No single food contains all the essential nutrients the body needs to be healthy and function efficiently. The nutritional value of a person's diet depends on the overall mixture or balance of foods that is eaten over a period of time as well as on the needs of the individual eating them. That is why a balanced diet is one that is likely to include a large number or variety of foods, so adequate intakes of all the nutrients are achieved.

Nutrients

We all need energy from foods to live. The main nutrients found in foods that provide energy are:

- protein
- fat
- carbohydrate.

Although not classified as a nutrient, alcohol also provides energy.

Some nutrients are essential for life though they are needed in only tiny amounts:

- vitamins
- minerals.

Vitamins and minerals do not provide energy.

Fibre does not provide us with energy, but is needed to keep our digestion working properly. It helps us to get rid of waste products from the body and keeps our bowels working properly.

Fluid is vital – without fluid we will not live for long. Adequate fluid is needed to keep us healthy. Water is the main fluid and does not provide energy.

Key points

- **We all need energy from foods to live.**
- **Protein, fat, carbohydrate and alcohol all provide energy.**
- **Vitamins and minerals are essential for life, but do not provide energy and are only needed in tiny amounts.**

Energy

We need energy for our bodies to function and be active. In the body, energy is used to maintain those activities that keep us alive. These include maintaining the body temperature, processes such as breathing, the beating of the heart, the blood circulating and the synthesis of the different body tissues – such as the growth of hair. The energy used in these processes is called the Basal Metabolic Rate (BMR).

All of physical activities – whether vigorous, such as running, or small, such as blinking – that use muscles also require energy.

Foods contain a mixture of nutrients – for example, whole milk contains a mixture of protein, fat (in the cream on top of the milk) as well as some carbohydrate (in the form of the sugar lactose). The protein, fat and carbohydrate all provide energy. Milk also contains other nutrients, such as calcium and vitamins, which do not provide energy. Milk also contains water.

Different foods provide different amounts of energy depending on the amounts of the various energy-providing nutrients they contain. Energy from food is measured in kilojoules (kJ) or kilocalories (kcal).

The energy provided by carbohydrate, protein, alcohol and fat in food and drinks is as follows:

The energy providers

1g carbohydrate provides 16 kJ (3.75 kcal)
1g protein provides 17 kJ (4 kcal)
1g alcohol provides 29 kJ (7 kcal)
1g of fat provides 37 kJ (9 kcal)

As a rough measure, 1 gram is the equivalent of a quarter of a level teaspoon.

Energy requirements

The amount of energy a person needs depends on a number of factors. These include body size and composition – that is, how tall and heavy a person is and how much lean tissue (muscle) they carry, compared with how much fat they carry. Muscle tissue uses up more energy than fat tissue. In general, females require less energy than males because females have a smaller body size, less muscle tissue and more fat than males. Guideline daily amounts (GDAs) for energy are 2,000 kcal for adult women and 2,500 kcal for adult men.

During the latter stage of pregnancy, however, a woman requires approximately 200 extra kcal (840 kJ) per day. When she is breastfeeding a baby of two months of age, however, she requires approximately 500 kcal (2,100 kJ) extra each day.

Energy requirements also depend on age and on how active a person is. Infants and children need energy for growth. Teenagers or adolescents in the age group 15–18 years of age often have the highest requirements for energy of any age group, as they are growing and also usually very active. In general, adults require less energy as they get older – elderly people typically have less muscle and are less active than younger adults.

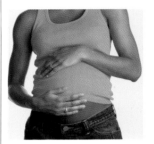

In the late stage of pregnancy women's energy requirements increase slightly

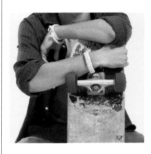

Teenagers have the highest energy requirements

 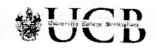

Introduction

We eat and ⌐ ⌐arent
that what we ⌐th our
immediate h

For example, if a perso
inadvertently consume
has been contaminate
could be in jeopardy. C
habitually eats a diet tl
quantities of a nutrien
deficiency that could le
future. Therefore, peop
only have a special res⌐
health of the consume
hygiene practices, but ⌐
future health of the po
food and healthier cho
products and dishes.

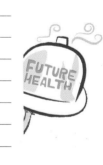

Recent government su⌐
identified that more ar
prepared and cooked o
reasons for this change
disposable income, inc⌐
busy lifestyles and so on. In addition to this, consumers are
increasingly interested in the effect of diet on health – as
reflected in the increasing number of reports and features
on food and diet in the media and consumer demands for
nutrition labelling on foods, etc. People whose work
involves food will be better placed to meet the needs of
consumers if they, themselves, have a good, basic
understanding of nutrition.

There in no legal responsibility to understand nutrition, but
a sound basic knowledge could stand you in good stead for
career opportunities, better job security, commercial
opportunities and financial gains by better understanding
the needs of consumers. You don't have to memorise
every detail of nutrition in this book, but you should
develop an understanding of its contents and how to use it
as a source of reference.

Chapter 1
An introduction to nutrition

If you eat a variety of foods, in adequate amounts, you will receive sufficient nutrients to stay healthy.

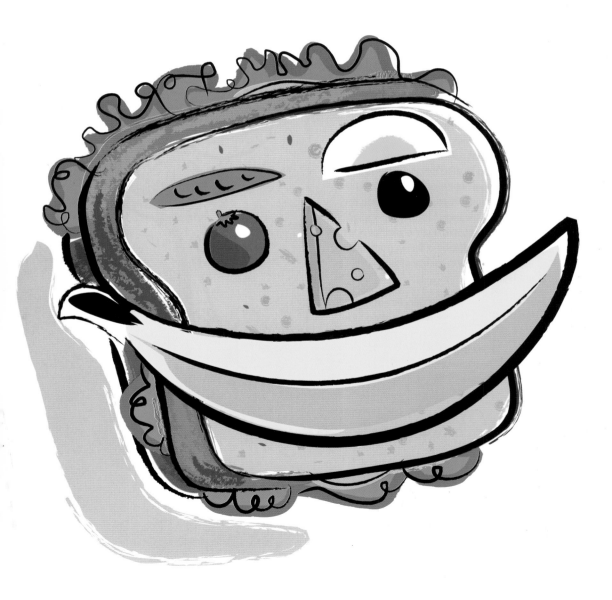

The table below shows the average energy cost of some different activities. People with sedentary jobs (such as office workers) use up less energy than people with physically-demanding jobs (such as plasterers and builders).

Examples of typical energy usage

Activity	Energy used up in 20 minutes by an adult woman
Sleeping	67 kJ/16 kcal
Reading	84 kJ/20 kcal
Driving	125 kJ/30 kcal
Walking	335 kJ/80 kcal
Swimming	460 kJ/110 kcal
Jogging	586 kJ/140 kcal
Running fast	837 kJ/200 kcal

So we all need energy to live and energy is provided by the following nutrients:

- protein
- fat
- carbohydrate.

Key points

- Different foods provide different amounts of energy depending on the amounts of the various energy-providing nutrients they contain.
- The amount of energy a person needs depends on a number of factors: body size and composition, whether they are male or female, how physically active they are and their age.

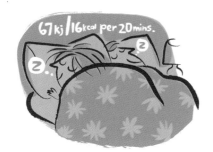

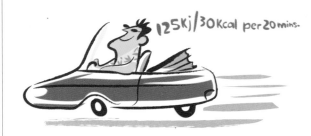

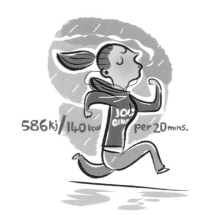

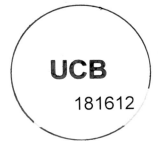

Protein

The human body is made up of cells. These cells vary in their makeup and are grouped together to make all of the vital organs of the body – such as the liver, heart or skin – as well as red and white blood cells. As the cells of the body die, they are replaced as part of a continuing cycle of renewal – for example, red blood cells are replaced approximately every 120 days.

Proteins are essential constituents of all cells, where they regulate body processes or provide structure. Protein must be provided in the diet for the growth of new cells – such as occurs in children or the foetus of a pregnant woman. Proteins are also needed for repair of the body cells. Any excess protein that is not needed for growth or repair is used to provide energy.

Protein foods are those foods that contain a large proportion of protein. They can be divided into animal sources and plant sources.

Animal sources of protein include:

- meat
- poultry
- offal
- fish
- eggs
- milk and dairy foods like cheese and yoghurt.

Plant sources of protein include:

- soya and soya foods
- pulses such as beans, lentils, peas
- nuts.

A small amount of protein is also provided by bread, other cereals like breakfast cereals and pasta as well as potatoes.

Proteins consist of chains of amino acids – these are the basic, tiny building blocks from which proteins are made.

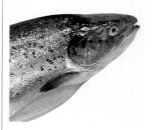

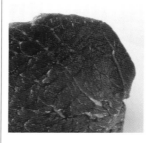

Animal sources of protein include fish and meat

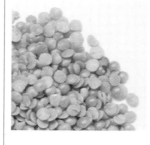

Plant sources of protein include pulses

Amino acids can be divided into two types:

- **essential** (indispensable)

- **non-essential** (dispensable).

Indispensable amino acids cannot be made in the body in amounts sufficient for health and must, therefore, be present in the diet. Dispensable amino acids are equally necessary as components of proteins in the body, but they can be made within the body.

Eating the right mix of food at each meal will provide a balance of indispensable and dispensable amino acids. Mixtures of plant protein foods – such as, beans on toast – complement each other as most plant protein foods provide insufficient amounts of at least one indispensable amino acid.

On average, adults in the UK eat around 50g of protein per day of which about one third comes from plant sources – such as vegetables, breakfast cereals and bread – and two thirds from animal sources, such as meat, milk, eggs, fish and cheese. Vegetarians should eat a wide range of plant proteins to make sure they get an adequate mix of all the amino acids.

The amount of protein we need changes during a lifetime. Infants, children and adolescents need protein for growth. Adults need protein for tissue maintenance and repair. Pregnant women need extra protein for the growth of their babies and women who are breastfeeding need protein to produce breast milk.

Key points

- Proteins are essential constituents of all cells – we need different amounts of protein during life for growth, tissue maintenance and repair.

- Proteins can be provided by animal sources and plant sources.

- Proteins consist of chains of amino acids.

- Eating the right mix of food is important to provide the right balance of essential (indispensable) and non-essential (dispensable) amino acids.

Fat

Fats provide the body with energy in a concentrated form as they provide 9 kcal (37 kJ) per g. They are also needed to help absorb some of the fat-soluble vitamins.

Sources of fat include 'visible fats' (those that can easily be seen) such as butter, margarine and other, cooking fats and oils and the fat on meat. There are also the 'invisible fats' (those that cannot easily be seen) – that is, fat in foods such as cheese, biscuits and cakes, pies and pastries and nuts.

The components of fat are known as fatty acids, of which there are three main classes:

- saturated fatty acids (saturates) – have the most stable structure and are mainly solid at room temperature

- monounsaturated fatty acids (monounsaturates) – are less stable and are liquid at room temperature

- polyunsaturated fatty acids (polyunsaturates) – are also liquid at room temperature and are the most prone to reacting with oxygen in the air and becoming rancid.

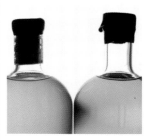

Sources of fat include visible and invisible fats

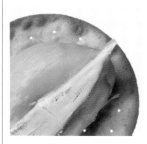

All food fats are a mixture of the three types listed above, although the proportions of each vary – for example, saturated fats are found mainly in foods such as lard, hard margarine and butter. However, coconut oil and palm oil also contain predominantly saturated fatty acids. Olive oil and rapeseed oil contain mainly monounsaturates. Sunflower oil, corn oil and soya oil contain mainly polyunsaturated fatty acids.

Oil-rich fish – such as mackerel, sardines, salmon, herrings and trout – are rich sources of a particular family of polyunsaturates known as n-3 fatty acids (also called omega 3 fatty acids or fish oils). These fatty acids are important as they have an anti-inflammatory effect, which is helpful for keeping joints pain free from arthritis and preventing coronary heart disease.

Fat is important for health, but only in small amounts. No more than 35 % of the energy in our diets should come from fat and no more than 11 % of energy should come from saturates. Although substantial reductions in total fat intake have been achieved in recent years, most people still consume too many saturates in their diets.

GDAs for fats are 70g for women and 95g for men. GDAs for saturated fats are 20g for women and 30g for men.

Diets that are high in fat, particularly the saturates, are linked with an increased risk of heart disease through their effect on blood cholesterol levels. High-fat diets (due to their high energy content) may also cause weight gain, if physical activity levels and hence energy expenditure is lower than energy intake.

Key points

- Fats provide the body with energy in a concentrated form.

- Fat is important for health, but only in small amounts.

- Most people still consume too many saturates in their diets and diets rich in the saturated fatty acids are linked with an increased risk of heart disease.

Carbohydrates

There are three major groups of carbohydrates in food:

- starches
- sugars
- fibre.

Starches and sugar are a major source of food energy for people throughout the world. At least half the energy in the diet should come from carbohydrate, the majority of which should come from starch. Fibre does not provide energy, but is important for bowel health.

Starches

Starch forms the major energy reserve of most plants, where it is stored in the tubers (for example in potatoes), roots (such as in parsnips) and seeds (such as of the grains of cereals like oats, rice and wheat) of plants. The principal sources of starch in the UK diet are wheat (such as found in bread, breakfast cereals, pasta and cous-cous), rice, other cereals (such as maize and oats) and potatoes.

Sugars

The principal sources of sugars in the UK diet are table sugar (sucrose), which is derived from sugar cane and sugar beet. Glucose syrups are used in cakes, biscuits, sports drinks and confectionery. These types of sugar are termed non-milk extrinsic sugars (NMES) because they are an added ingredient rather than an integral part of a foodstuff. Other sources of sugar in the diet are milk (lactose), fruit (fructose) where the sugar component is part of the food.

Consuming a lot of certain types of sugar-containing foods and drinks (those containing NMES) at frequent intervals, especially between meals, is associated with increased risk of tooth decay (dental caries). The type of sugar present and where it is found in a food affect its ability to cause dental caries. Lactose, for example, is not associated with dental caries when consumed in the form of dairy products. It is the NMES that are most strongly associated with increased risk of dental caries. The effect of sugar can be lessened by regular brushing of teeth (twice daily for two minutes) and the use of fluoride toothpaste.

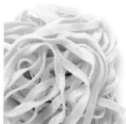

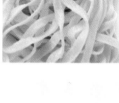

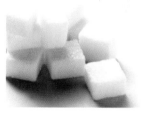

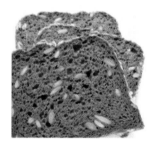

The three major groups of carbohydrates in food are starches, sugars and fibre

Fibre

Fibre used to be called roughage and is found in most cereal foods such as bread and breakfast cereals. It is found particularly in the wholegrain varieties like wholemeal bread, wholegrain breakfast cereals, brown rice and brown pasta. It is also found in pulses (beans and lentils), fruit and vegetables. Fibre makes up the components from plant foods that generally cannot be absorbed into the body. Some fibre constituents (mainly those from the cereals like wheat) add bulk to the faeces, which is important for bowel health and in preventing constipation. Other fibre constituents, found in fruit, vegetables, pulses and oats can help to reduce the amount of cholesterol in the blood by reducing absorption. However, eating very large amounts of fibre can decrease the absorption of some minerals.

On average we eat only about 12g of fibre a day. It has been recommended that we should aim to eat at least 18g per day to prevent problems like constipation, piles (haemorrhoids) and bowel cancer. Most of the fibre eaten comes from potatoes, cereal products (like bread and breakfast cereals) and vegetables.

Key points

- There are three major groups of carbohydrates in food: starches, sugars and fibre.

- Starches and sugars provide energy. Fibre does not, but it is important for bowel health.

- At least half the energy in the diet should come from carbohydrate, the majority of which should come from starch.

- Eating a lot of certain types of sugar-containing foods and drinks, especially between meals, is associated with increased risk of tooth decay.

Vitamins

Vitamins are complex substances needed in very tiny amounts for many different body processes. Vitamins have numerous functions in the body but, as they cannot be made in the body, they must be provided by diet. There are two main groups of vitamins:

■ **fat-soluble vitamins**, which are found in fatty foods e.g. vitamin A and D in butter, and can be stored in the body

■ **water-soluble vitamins**, which are found in foods that contain amounts of water such as fruit and vegetables, and cannot be stored in the body so a regular supply is required in the diet.

The table below gives the main functions and sources of each vitamin.

Vitamin functions and sources

Fat-soluble vitamins

Vitamin	Main functions	Sources
A (retinol and beta carotene)	Maintains and repairs tissues needed for growth and development. Essential for immune function, normal and night vision.	Milk, cheese, eggs, liver, oily fish. Beta carotene (and other carotenoids): vegetables and fruit, especially carrots, tomatoes, mangoes, apricots and green leafy vegetables.
D	Promotes calcium absorption from food. Essential for bones and teeth.	Sunshine, fortified margarines and breakfast cereals, meat, oily fish, eggs.
E	Acts as an antioxidant, protects cell membranes from damage by oxygen.	Vegetable oils, margarines, wholegrain cereals, nuts, green leafy vegetables.
K	Essential for blood clotting.	Dark green leafy vegetables, fruit, vegetable oils, cereals, meat.

Water-soluble vitamins

Vitamin	Main functions	Sources
C	Needed for the production of collagen, which is used in the structure of connective tissue of skin, muscles and blood vessel walls and also for bones. Helps wound healing and iron absorption. Acts as an antioxidant.	Fruits, especially citrus fruits, fruit juices, green vegetables, salad, potatoes, peppers, kiwi fruit.
B_1	Involved in the release of energy from carbohydrate. Important for brain and nerves.	Cereals, nuts, pulses, green vegetables, pork, fruits, fortified breakfast cereals.
B_2	Involved in energy release, especially from fat and protein.	Liver, milk, cheese, yogurt, eggs, green vegetables, yeast extract, fortified breakfast cereals.
Niacin	Involved in the release of energy.	Liver, beef, pork, lamb, fish, fortified breakfast cereals and other cereal products.
B_{12}	Necessary for the proper formation of blood cells and nerve fibres.	Offal, meat, eggs, fish, milk, fortified breakfast cereals. No plant foods contain a source of B_{12} that the body can absorb naturally.
Folate (folic acid)	Involved in the formation of blood cells. Reduces risk of neural tube defects in early pregnancy such as spina bifida.	Liver, orange juice, dark green vegetables, nuts, wholemeal bread, fortified breakfast cereals and bread.
B_6	Involved in the metabolism of protein.	Widely distributed in foods; potatoes, beef, fish, chicken, cereals.

Minerals

Minerals are essential for health and must be derived from food. Minerals are needed in relatively small amounts and for a variety of body functions. The table below gives the main functions and sources of each mineral.

Mineral functions and sources

Mineral	Main functions	Sources
Calcium	Has a structural role in bones and teeth. Also essential for cellular structure. It assists muscle contractions to occur.	Milk and milk products, bread, pulses, green vegetables, dried fruits, nuts, seeds, soft bones found in canned fish such as sardines.
Magnesium	Involved in skeletal development, nerve and muscle function. It is also necessary for the functioning of some enzymes involved in energy use.	Cereals, particularly wholegrain and wholemeal products, nuts, seeds, green vegetables, milk, meat, potatoes.
Phosphorus	Has a structural role in bones and teeth. Also a constituent of all the major classes of a number of substances in the body.	Milk, milk products, bread, meat and poultry.
Sodium	Involved in maintaining the water balance of the body and is also essential for muscle and nerve activity. However, a high sodium intake has been linked to increased blood pressure. Most people eat too much sodium.	Processed foods: bread, cereal products, breakfast cereals, meat products, pickles, canned vegetables, canned and packet sauces and soups, packet snack foods, spreading fats, cheese and salt added to food.
Potassium	Complements and counterbalances the action of sodium.	Vegetables, potatoes, fruit, especially bananas, juices, bread, fish, nuts, seeds.
Iron	Important for the formation of red blood cells. Meat and meat products are a rich source of well-absorbed iron.	Plant sources of iron are cereals, bread, breakfast cereals, green leafy vegetables, beans, lentils and dried fruit. To help absorption from plant sources, a source of vitamin C should be consumed at the same meal as the iron-containing food.
Zinc	Involved in the metabolism of protein, carbohydrates and fats, and formation of cells in the immune system.	Meat, meat products, milk, milk products, bread, cereal products, especially wholemeal, eggs, beans, lentils, nuts, sweetcorn, rice.
Copper	A component of a number of enzymes.	Shellfish, liver, meat, bread, cereal products, vegetables, tap water.
Selenium	Acts as an antioxidant by being an integral part of one of the enzymes that protects against oxidative damage.	Nuts, especially Brazil nuts, cereals, meat, particularly offal, fish, particularly shellfish.
Iodine	A key part of the thyroid hormones that help control metabolic rate, cellular metabolism and integrity of connective tissue.	Fish, seaweed, milk, milk products, beer, meat products.
Fluoride	Protects against tooth decay and has a role in bone mineralisation.	Fish, water, tea.

Active substances found in plant foods

Plenty of fruit and vegetables and other plant foods are recommended in our diets because they provide important vitamins, minerals and fibre and are generally low in fat. In addition, they contain active substances (antioxidants) that may have health benefits such as keeping cells healthy and preventing damage. Research has shown that eating plenty of fruit and vegetables and other plant foods can help to lower the risk of some diseases – such as heart disease and cancer – due to some part to the, as yet unknown, actions of these active compounds.

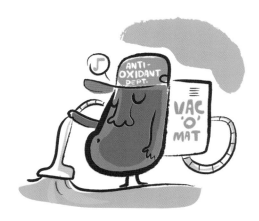

The immune system

The system in the body that helps the resistance to infections and the early stages of diseases is called the immune system. As described, certain nutrients such as zinc and vitamin C help the immune system to work efficiently.

Key points

- Vitamins and minerals cannot be made in the body so must be provided by food.

- Plant foods contain active substances (antioxidants) that may have health benefits such as keeping cells healthy and preventing damage.

- Some nutrients help the immune system to work efficiently.

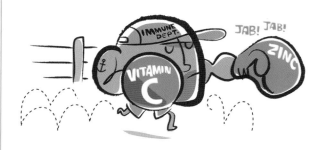

Eating a mixed diet

All foods provide energy and nutrients and it is achieving the correct intake of nutrients that is important for health.

Hardly any foods provide only one nutrient. Most are very complex mixtures, consisting mainly of carbohydrates, fats and proteins together with water and a selection of vitamins and minerals. For example, 100g of raw potato provides about 17g carbohydrate, 2g of protein, 80g of water and less than 0.5g of vitamins and minerals. If the potatoes are fried as chips, they will also provide some fat.

Different foods provide different vitamins and minerals – therefore a healthy diet should include a variety of foods. For example, dairy products such as milk and yoghurt, are good sources of calcium, but they contain very little vitamin C. Citrus fruits are good sources of vitamin C, but they do not provide any iron and so on. The important message is to eat a balanced and varied diet.

Typical nutritional breakdown of a potato:

1. water
2. carbohydrate
3. protein
4. vitamins and minerals

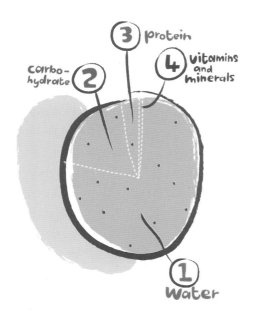

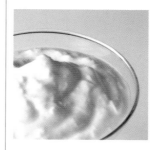

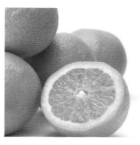

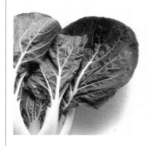

A healthy diet should include a variety of foods

Other food constituents

Water

Water comprises about two-thirds of the body's weight, and is necessary for all body processes to take place. The need for water by the body is second only to its need for air to breathe – adults can survive for many weeks without food, but only a few days without water. Water comes from solid foods, which contain a proportion of water, with such items as fruit and vegetables containing significant amounts of fluid, as well as drinks. Fluid is lost through breathing (being lost in the exhaled air) and sweating as well as in urine. The kidneys regulate the balance of water retained in the body. Most people need 1.2 litres (three pints or six to eight cups) of fluid per day from food and drinks.

Additives

Additives are used to give foods flavour, colour and texture, as well as preserving them and making them safe to eat for longer. Additives must be tested before being approved for use in small amounts in certain foods. An E number shows that a food additive has been approved for use in the European Community.

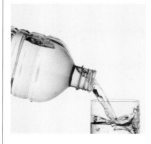

Drink 1.2 litres of water a day

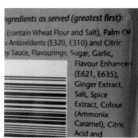

Additives can only be used in small amounts in certain foods

Key points

- Most foods provide a complex mixture of nutrients.

- A healthy diet should, therefore, consist of a variety of foods.

- Most people need 1.2 litres of fluid a day.

- Additives are used in small amounts to give food flavour, colour and texture. An E number shows that the food additive has been approved for use in the European community.

Summary

1. We all need energy from foods to live.

2. Protein, fat, carbohydrate and alcohol all provide energy.

3. Vitamins and minerals are essential for life, but do not provide energy and are only needed in only tiny amounts.

4. Different foods provide different amounts of energy depending on the amounts of the various energy-providing nutrients they contain.

5. The amount of energy a person needs depends on a number of factors: body size and composition, whether they are male or female, how physically active they are and their age.

6. Proteins are essential constituents of all cells – we need different amounts of protein during life for growth, tissue maintenance and repair.

7. Proteins can be provided by animal sources and plant sources.

8. Proteins consist of chains of amino acids.

9. Eating the right mix of food is important to provide the right balance of essential (indispensable) and non-essential (dispensable) amino acids.

10. Fats provide the body with energy in a concentrated form.

11. Fat is important for health, but only in small amounts.

12. Most people consume too many saturates in their diets and diets rich in the saturated fatty acids are linked with an increased risk of heart disease.

13. There are three major groups of carbohydrates in food: starches, sugars and fibre.

14. Starches and sugars provide energy. Fibre does not, but it is important for bowel health.

15. At least half the energy in the diet should come from carbohydrate, the majority of which should come from starch.

16. Eating a lot of certain types of sugar-containing foods and drinks, especially between meals, is associated with increased risk of tooth decay.

17. Vitamins and minerals cannot be made in the body so must be provided by food.

18. Plant foods contain active substances (antioxidants) that may have health benefits such as keeping cells healthy and preventing damage.

19. Some vitamins help the immune system to work efficiently.

20. Most foods provide a complex mixture of nutrients.

21. A healthy diet should, therefore, consist of a variety of foods.

22. Most people need 1.2 litres of fluid a day.

23. Additives are used in small amounts to give food flavour, colour and texture. An E number shows that the food additive has been approved for use in the European community.

Chapter 2
The nutrient content of foods

Almost all food must be processed in some way before it can be eaten and each process will have an impact on the nutrient content. This chapter looks at the effect of processing on the nutrient content of the food and ways of minimising nutrient loss. Nutrients lost during processing may be replaced and some common foods are fortified. There are rules governing the fortification of food, nutrition labelling and nutrition claims. Some rules are mandatory and others are voluntary.

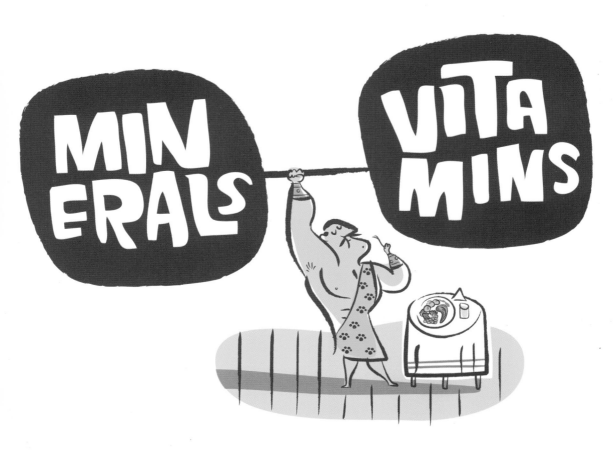

Nutrient loss and the fortification of foods

Nutrients, such as vitamins and minerals, can be added to foods during processing and production. Food components, such as fibre, may also be added to some foods. Adding nutrients and other components to foods particularly staple foods, such as flour and other cereal products, can increase intakes of certain vitamins and minerals among the whole population.

Nutrients or food components may be added for a variety of reasons. Nutrients lost during food processing may be replaced. This is particularly important if the food was a good source of the nutrient before processing. For example, it is UK law that the nutrients removed with the bran (the outer part of the wheat grain which contains most of the fibre as well as certain vitamins and minerals) during the milling of wheat to make all flour, except wholemeal, must be replaced. Therefore the B vitamins B_1 (thiamin) and niacin, and also calcium and iron are added to white flour.

Nutrients may be added to foods in amounts greater than would normally be present. This is known as 'food fortification'. Nutrients should not be added in large amounts that could be harmful to people eating their usual quantity of food. Fortification can be either mandatory or voluntary. Commonly fortified foods in the UK include white flour, margarine, infant formulae milks, which are fortified by law, and breakfast cereals and spreads (such as low fat spreads) for which fortification is voluntary.

UK law states that margarine must be fortified with vitamins A and D. This is not because they are lost during processing but because many people use margarine instead of butter, which is a source of these nutrients. Average intakes of vitamin D would drop considerably if margarine was not fortified, and some people could be at risk of low intakes. This is especially true of people with less exposure to sunlight, such as children, older people and those that live in the most northern parts of the UK. Fortifying margarine with vitamin A is important because some people have low intakes, particularly those who do not eat good sources of vitamin A such as full-cream milk and dairy products, liver, oily fish, eggs and carrots and

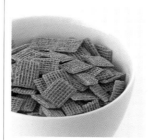

Many breakfast cereals are fortified with vitamins and minerals

other orange or red coloured items such as apricots, tomatoes and mangoes. Reduced- and low-fat spreads are usually also fortified with vitamin A and D, but this is done voluntarily by the manufacturers.

Many breakfast cereals are fortified voluntarily with vitamins and minerals such as B vitamins, folic acid and iron.

When nutrients are added to foods, manufacturers may be able to make a claim on the label that the food is a good source of the nutrient or food component – for example, white bread with added fibre can be labelled 'high in fibre'.

Foods that are produced for vegans, such as soya products, are often fortified with vitamin B_{12}. As foods from plant sources do not contain this vitamin, fortified foods are the main dietary source of vitamin B_{12} for vegans. Some soya milk substitutes are also fortified with calcium.

Many manufactured foods for infants are fortified with iron and vitamin D.

Other foods, such as meal replacements, sports drinks and slimming products, may be fortified with a range of vitamins and minerals.

Fortification is, therefore, commonplace in the UK and consideration is being given to whether guidance or regulations should be in place to limit the quantities of nutrients that can be added to foods to avoid the risk of excess intakes.

Key points

- Nutrients, such as vitamins and minerals, and other components, such as fibre, can be added to foods during processing and production.

- When nutrients are added to foods in amounts greater than would normally be present, this is known as 'food fortification'.

- Fortification can be either mandatory or voluntary.

- When nutrients or components are added to foods, manufacturers may be able to make claims on the food labels – such as 'high in calcium' or 'high in fibre'.

Preventing loss of nutrients

Many factors influence the nutrient content of foods including storage, processing, cooking and preservation. Most foods have to be prepared and cooked before they can be eaten. For some foods the process may be simple, as in the peeling of an orange. For others it may be complicated – for example, wheat grains must be separated from the inedible parts of the plant (the outer bran) and milled into flour, which in turn has to be treated before being baked into bread. At each stage, some of the nutrients can be lost. The nutrient levels of a food may be further reduced if the food is stored for long periods, particularly if conditions are not ideal.

These losses, although not critical if a good mixed diet is eaten, should be kept to a minimum.

Cooking

The heat of cooking causes chemical and physical changes in food that make the raw product palatable and digestible and may aid its preservation. Cooking, however, often results in the loss of nutrients – this is greatest at high temperatures and over long cooking times or if an excessive amount of liquid is used.

The water-soluble vitamins are particularly vulnerable during the process of cooking. The losses of vitamins and minerals are reduced if the cooking water is not discarded but used in, for example, soups and gravies.

The effects of microwaves and infra-red cooking on nutrients are similar to the effects of the cooking methods they replace. When used for reheating, they cause little additional destruction of nutrients.

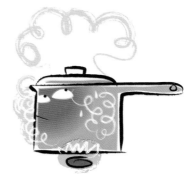

Preservation

Freezing is a popular method of food preservation that can result in the loss of vitamin B_1 (thiamin) and vitamin C when vegetables are blanched by quickly immersing in hot water before freezing. This loss is, however, less than would otherwise result from the continuing action of enzymes in the plant tissues during storage. These enzymes can break down plant tissues and cause deterioration of the food. Freezing inhibits the actions of these enzymes. If frozen foods are kept below −18°C for a year, there is little further loss of nutritional value until the food is thawed. In general, there is little difference between the nutrient content of cooked fresh foods and cooked frozen foods.

Heat processing in metal cans or bottling in glass jars is undertaken to preserve foods by destroying micro-organisms (bacteria) which cause food to rot or perish. The process will also reduce the amounts of heat-sensitive vitamins, especially B_1 (thiamin), folate and vitamin C. The losses will depend on the length of time needed to destroy any micro-organisms and also to cook the food. These losses will be greater for larger cans and in foods that are solid, such as ham, because of the slow transfer of heat from the outside to the centre. Losses will also depend on the acidity of the food and the presence of light and air.

Dehydration in carefully controlled conditions has little effect on most nutrients, but destroys about half of the vitamin C. Vitamin B_1 (thiamin) is completely lost if sulphur dioxide is added as a preservative such as can occur in fruit products (dried apricots) and items like sausages. Prolonged sun drying, as in the production of raisins, allows substantial changes to occur. Suitable packaging of dried foods is essential to prevent nutrient losses during extended storage.

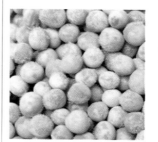

Some vitamins can be lost if vegetables are blanched before freezing

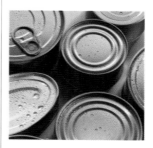

Heat processing may result in nutrient loss if heat is applied too long

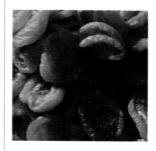

In carefully controlled conditions, dehydration has little effect on most nutrients

Key points

- The loss of nutrients associated with cooking is greatest at high temperatures and over a long time, or if an excessive amount of liquid is used.

- Various techniques can be used to preserve the nutrient content and quality of food – for example, freezing, canning, dehydration.

Stability of individual nutrients

Protein is changed (in a process called denaturisation) by heat and when heating is severe it becomes less available for utilisation in the body. This is partly because the changes in structure make the protein more difficult to digest and partly because some of the component amino acids are changed.

Vitamin A (both in the forms of retinol and beta-carotene) are stable throughout most cooking procedures, although at high temperatures (such as occur in canning) losses occur. There are also losses during prolonged storage if light and air are not rigorously excluded.

The B vitamins are all water-soluble and most are sensitive to heat.

Vitamin B_1 (thiamin) is one of the least stable vitamins. It is readily dissolved out of foods into the cooking water and is easily lost in the juices from meat. It is fairly stable when heated if the food is acid, but the losses can be considerable under alkaline conditions, especially if sodium bicarbonate is added during cooking. It has been calculated that, on average, 20 % of the thiamin content of all food brought into the home is lost during cooking and reheating, but the loss is greater in some foods than others. Any foods that have been preserved by the use of sulphur dioxide, such as sausages, wine and some potato products, will contain very little thiamin.

Riboflavin can be lost in discarded cooking water and meat juices – it is also unstable to alkali and especially sensitive to light (and so is lost from milk if a bottle is left on a doorstep).

Niacin is an exceptionally stable vitamin and will be lost only through its solubility in water.

Other B-vitamins are all soluble in water. Vitamin B_6, folate and pantothenic acid are also sensitive to heat and can therefore be lost to some extent in cooking and canning.

Vitamin C is the least stable of all the vitamins. In addition to being water-soluble, it is very readily destroyed by air in a process called oxidation. The destruction of vitamin C is accelerated by heat, by alkali and by the presence of certain metals, e.g. copper and iron. Vitamin C is also rapidly oxidised when an enzyme present in fruit and vegetables is released by any physical damage to the plant, such as cutting or bruising. Finely chopping food rather than leaving it in whole pieces can cause greater losses of vitamin C. Poor cooking practices such as prolonged boiling of green vegetables in large amounts of water, followed by keeping them hot, can result in the destruction of all the vitamin C originally present. Vitamin C is, however, partly protected by sulphur dioxide.

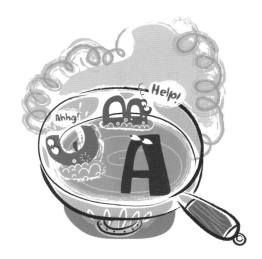

Key point

- If food is carefully prepared and correctly stored, the overall loss of vitamins and minerals need not be significant.

Nutrition information on food labels

Many food labels have nutrition information on them. This can help consumers to find out the amount of different nutrients in the foods they eat. It can also help them to select foods that are, for example, lower in fat or higher in fibre than other products.

Food manufacturers are not obliged by law to give nutrition information unless they make a nutrition claim – for example, 'low fat' or 'high fibre' – but if they do, they must follow certain rules. If they choose to provide nutrition information, it must be given for 100g or 100 ml of the product in one of two formats: the 'Big 4' and 'Big 4 and Little 4' (see opposite).

Information can also be given per serving or per portion, provided that the number of portions is stated.

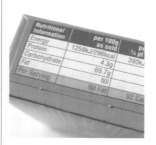

Big 4

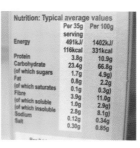

Big 4 and Little 4

Key points

- Food manufacturers are not obliged by law to give nutrition information unless they make a nutrition claim.

- If a claim is made, such as 'low in fat' or 'high in fibre', manufactures must be provided nutrition information in one of two forms – the 'Big 4' or the 'Big 4 and Little 4'.

Nutrition claims

Consumers can use nutrient claims as a quick guide to the content of a product. Claims usually use such terms as 'low', 'high' and 'source of'. Claims can be used for fortified foods, foods that are naturally high in different nutrients and also foods that have been modified to contain less of a certain nutrient. If a manufacturer makes a claim about a nutrient, nutrition information must be provided on the label.

Government guidelines have been issued for standards that must be met if certain claims are made.

For example:

Low fat = no more than 3g of fat per 100g or per serving (whichever is the greater)

High in fibre = more than 6g of fibre per 100g or per serving

Manufacturers are not allowed to state or imply that a food can prevent, treat or cure a disease, such as heart disease.

Many manufacturers and retailers have adopted the Food Standards Agency's 'traffic light' labelling. This system is designed to show, at a glance, if the food has high, medium or low amounts of fat, saturated fat, sugars and salt. The label also shows how much of each nutrient is in a portion so, if two labels have the same colour, you can compare the figures and choose the one that is lower to make a healthier choice.

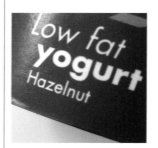

If a nutrient claim is made, nutritional information must be provided on the label

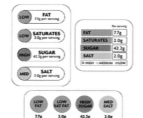

Traffic light labelling is designed to show, at a glance, if the food has high, medium or low amounts of fat, saturated fat, sugars and salt

Key points

- If a manufacturer makes a claim about a nutrient, nutrition information must be provided on the label.

- Manufacturers are not allowed to state or imply that a food can prevent, treat or cure a disease.

- Many manufacturers and retailers have adopted the Food Standards Agency's 'traffic light' labelling, designed to show, at a glance, if the food has high, medium or low amounts of fat, saturated fat, sugars and salt and how much of each nutrient is in a portion.

Summary

1. Nutrients, such as vitamins and minerals, and other components, such as fibre, can be added to foods during processing and production.

2. When nutrients are added to foods in amounts greater than would normally be present, this is known as 'food fortification'.

3. Fortification can be either mandatory or voluntary.

4. When nutrients or components are added to foods, manufacturers may be able to make claims on the food labels – such as 'high in calcium' or 'high in fibre'.

5. The loss of nutrients associated with cooking is greatest at high temperatures and over a long time, or if an excessive amount of liquid is used.

6. Various techniques can be used to preserve the nutrient content and quality of food – for example, freezing, canning, dehydration.

7. If food is carefully prepared and correctly stored, the overall loss of vitamins and minerals need not be significant.

8. Food manufacturers are not obliged by law to give nutrition information unless they make a nutrition claim.

9. If a claim is made, such as 'low in fat' or 'high in fibre', manufacturers must provided nutrition information in one of two forms – the 'Big 4' or the 'Big 4 and Little 4'.

10. If a manufacturer makes a claim about a nutrient, nutrition information must be provided on the label.

11. Manufacturers are not allowed to state or imply that a food can prevent, treat or cure a disease.

12. Many manufacturers and retailers have adopted the Food Standards Agency's 'traffic light' labelling, designed to show, at a glance, if the food has high, medium or low amounts of fat, saturated fat, sugars and salt and how much of each nutrient is in a portion.

Chapter 3
Diet and health

The eatwell plate is a visual tool that illustrates the proportion and types of foods needed to make up a balanced diet. It is because of the scientifically established link between diet and disease that successive governments have been concerned to set dietary targets and recommendations. Improving the diet of the nation can have a significant impact on the health of the nation. Caterers can have a major influence on their customer's health by providing a range of healthy food options.

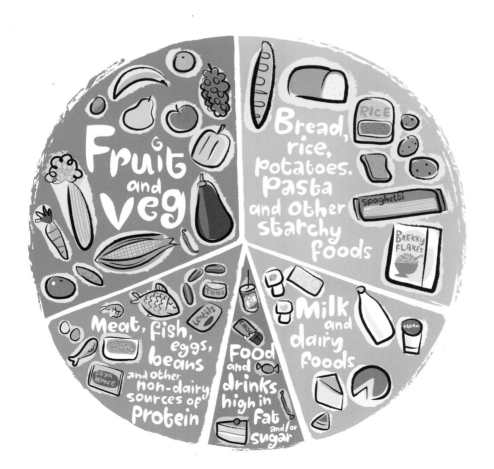

The eatwell plate

We need energy to live, but the balance between carbohydrate, fat and protein must be right for us to remain healthy. As already described the best source of energy is starchy carbohydrate foods. Too little protein can interfere with growth and other body functions, too much fat can lead to obesity and heart disease. Adequate intakes of vitamins, minerals and dietary fibre are important for health and there is growing evidence that a number of non-nutrient substances found in fruit and vegetables, are also important in promoting good health.

The concept of balance is presented as the illustrated guide of the eatwell plate, which shows the proportion and types of foods needed to make up a healthy diet.

The plate is divided into five food groups:

- fruit and vegetables
- bread, rice, potatoes, pasta and other starchy foods
- meat, fish, eggs, beans and other non-dairy sources of protein
- milk and dairy foods
- foods and drinks high in fat and/or sugar.

As can be seen the segments at the top of the plate which represent fruit and vegetables and the one for bread, rice, potatoes, pasta and other starchy foods are the largest and so these foods should be eaten in the largest amounts. The segment for foods and drinks high in fat and/or sugar is the smallest one as a large amount of these foods and drinks can be associated with ill health. Therefore these foods and drinks can be eaten in small amounts to add variety as part of a healthy diet.

The guide is shaped like a dinner plate to make it simple to understand.

Fruit and vegetables

All fruits and vegetables count except for potatoes, which are classed as a starchy food. The fruits and vegetables do not need to be fresh or raw – canned, dried, frozen and juiced are just as good. It is recommended that at least five portions are eaten per day. Fruit juice counts only as one portion however much is consumed in a day as the fibre is lost in making juices. The same rule applies to beans and pulses – e.g. baked beans – because vitamins are lost when beans and pulses are dried. Fruits and vegetables are low in fat and high in fibre so help to achieve the right balance between the nutrients in the diet.

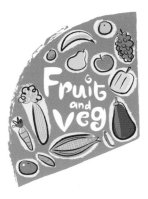

Bread, rice, potatoes, pasta and other starchy foods

Eating more starchy foods such as bread, rice, potatoes, and pasta will help to increase the amount of fibre in the diet and can also reduce the amount of fat eaten as these foods are filling and contain little fat. Changing the balance of the amounts of starchy carbohydrate and fat can be achieved at each meal, for example by having more rice or pasta with less sauce. These starchy foods should be a main part of most meals.

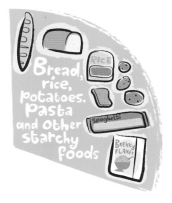

Meat, fish, eggs, beans and other non-dairy sources of protein

This group includes nuts, pulses and soya products, as well as meat (and poultry as well as offal like liver and kidney) fish, eggs and beans. These foods are rich in protein and other essential nutrients, such as iron, zinc, vitamin B_{12} and vitamin A. All visible fat and skin should be trimmed from meat and poultry and cooking methods should be employed that do not add fat – for example, grilling instead of frying. The size of this segment is smaller than for both fruit and vegetables and for bread, rice, potatoes, pasta and other starchy foods, indicating that only moderate amounts of these foods should be included in the diet.

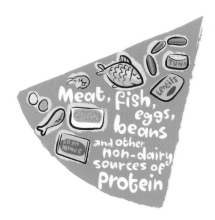

Milk and dairy foods

Milk and dairy foods are rich in calcium, protein and B vitamins. Whole milk, yoghurt and cheese also provide some vitamin A. As with meat, fish, eggs, beans and other non-dairy sources of protein the size of this segment is smaller than for both fruit and vegetables and for bread, rice, potatoes, pasta and other starchy foods, indicating that only moderate amounts of these foods should be included in the diet. For most people in the UK, milk and dairy foods are the most important sources of calcium in the diet. Calcium from milk is better absorbed in the body than from many other sources. Calcium is important for developing and maintaining strong teeth and bones. Choosing lower fat versions of milk, such as skimmed or semi-skimmed milk and low-fat yoghurts or cheese, will also help reduce fat intake while maintaining the amount of calcium taken.

For those who cannot take milk, soya milk, which has added calcium, can be used instead.

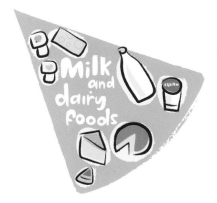

Foods and drinks high in fat and/or sugar

This group includes butter, margarine, spreading fats and cooking oils, which contain mainly fats. Snack foods such as crisps, sausage rolls, savoury pasties and onion bhajees all contain fat. Table sugar is included in this group as are items like soft drinks, jams, syrups, boiled sweets and jellies. Items such as cakes, pastries, desserts like ice creams and confectionery like chocolate and toffees and fudge, which all contain both fat and sugar, are also part of this group. This group forms the smallest segment indicating that these foods and drinks can be a part of a balanced diet, but only in *small* amounts.

The eatwell plate applies to all people including those who are overweight, vegetarians and people from ethnic minority backgrounds. It does not, however, apply to children under two years of age.

It is not necessary to achieve this balance at each meal, but this guide can apply to the food eaten over a day or even a week. The amounts that should be consumed will vary with energy needs (based on age, sex and physical activity levels) and appetite. Dishes containing more than one food can also fit into the model. A pizza, for example, has a dough base with toppings. The dough base counts as a starchy food so having a thick base is a good idea. If the pizza is homemade, the topping could be made with a reduced fat cheese or less cheese and more tomato as well as other vegetable items such as onions and peppers. Including a side salad with the pizza would increase the amount of vegetables eaten and fruit, as dessert, could complete the meal.

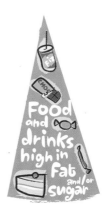

Key points

- No single food contains all the essential nutrients the body needs to be healthy and function efficiently.

- The eatwell plate shows the proportion and types of foods needed to make up a healthy diet.

- The guide is presented as a dinner plate so it is easy to understand.

- The plate is divided into five segments representing the proportions of five food groups:

  – fruit and vegetables

  – bread, rice, potatoes, pasta and other starchy foods

  – meat, fish, eggs, beans and other non-dairy sources of protein

  – milk and dairy foods

  – foods and drinks high in fat and/or sugar.

- It is not necessary to achieve this balance at each meal, but the eatwell plate can apply to the food eaten over a day or even a week.

Eight tips for eating well

The Government's eight tips for eating well are:

1. Base your meals on starchy foods

Starchy foods, such as bread, rice, breakfast cereals, pasta and potatoes, should make up about a third of the food we eat. They are a good source of energy and the main source of a range of nutrients in our diet. As well as starch, these foods contain fibre, calcium, iron and B vitamins. Wholegrain varieties should be included on a regular basis.

Some people think starchy foods are fattening, but gram for gram they contain less than half the calories of fat. You just need to watch the fats you add when cooking and serving these foods, because this is what increases the calorie content.

Wholegrain foods contain more fibre and other nutrients than white or refined starchy foods.

We also digest wholegrain foods more slowly so they can help make us feel full for longer.

Wholegrain foods include:

- wholemeal and wholegrain bread, pitta and chapatti
- wholewheat pasta and brown rice
- wholegrain breakfast cereals.

2. Eat lots of fruit and veg

It is important to include lots of different types of fruits and vegetables in the diet to provide vitamins, minerals and fibre as well as the protective antioxidants. A minimum of five portions of fruit and vegetables should be included in the diet everyday.

Most people know they should be eating more fruit and vegetables, but still aren't eating enough.

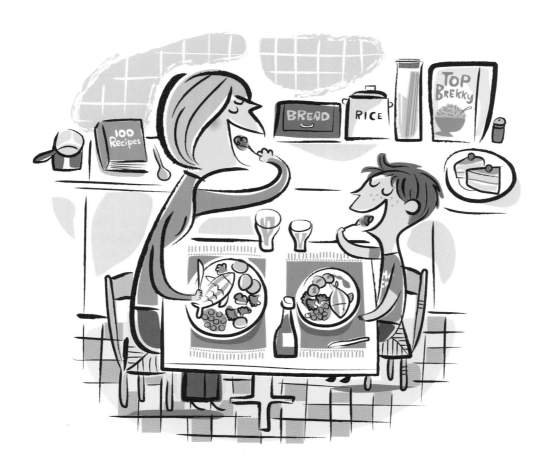

Try to eat at least five portions of a variety of fruit and vegetables every day. For example, you could have:

- a glass of juice and a sliced banana with your cereal at breakfast
- a side salad at lunch
- a pear as an afternoon snack
- a portion of peas or other vegetables with your evening meal.

You can choose from fresh, frozen, tinned, dried or juiced, but remember potatoes count as a starchy food, not as portions of fruit and vegetables.

3. Eat more fish
Most of us should be eating more fish. Aim for at least two portions each week – including a portion of oily fish. Fish is an excellent source of protein and contains many vitamins and minerals.

What are oily fish?
Some fish are called oily fish because they are rich in certain types of fats, called omega 3 fatty acids, which can help keep our hearts healthy.

How much oily fish?
Although most of us should be eating more oily fish, girls and women should have a maximum of 2 portions of oily fish a week (a portion is about 140g). And 4 is the recommended maximum number of portions for boys, men and older adults.

Examples of oily fish
Salmon, mackerel, trout, herring, fresh tuna, sardines, pilchards, eel.

Examples of white or non-oily fish
Cod, haddock, plaice, coley, tinned tuna, halibut, skate, sea bass, hake.

Shark, swordfish and marlin
Don't have more than one portion a week of these types of fish. This is because of the high levels of mercury in these fish.

4. Cut down on saturated fat and sugar
Avoid eating too many fried and fatty foods like cakes, biscuits and pastries. Choose lean meats and lower fat dairy products to help reduce your saturated fat intake.

Frequent consumption of sugary foods can increase the

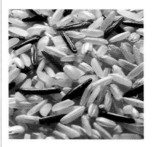

Eat starchy foods for dietary energy

risk of tooth decay, cut down of these foods and have them as part of meals rather than between meals. Many foods that contain added sugar can also be high in calories so cutting down could help you control your weight.

Foods high in saturated fat
Try to eat these sorts of foods less often or in small amounts:

- meat pies, sausages, meat with visible white fat
- hard cheese
- butter and lard
- pastry
- cakes and biscuits
- cream, soured cream and crème fraîche
- coconut oil, coconut cream or palm oil.

For a healthy choice, use just a small amount of vegetable oil or a reduced-fat spread instead of butter, lard or ghee. And when you are having meat, try to choose lean cuts and cut off any visible fat.

How do I know if a food is high in fat?
Some foods also give a figure for saturated fat, or 'saturates'. Use the following as a guide to what is a lot and what is a little fat per 100g of food.

This is **a lot** of fat:
20g fat or more per 100g
5g saturates or more per 100g

This is **a little** fat:
3g fat or less per 100g
1g saturates or less per 100g

If the amount of total fat is between 3g and 20g per 100g, this is a moderate amount of total fat. Between 1g and 5g of saturates is a moderate amount of saturated fat.

Try to choose more foods that only contain a little fat (3g fat or less per 100g) and cut down on foods that contain a lot of fat (20g fat or more per 100g).

How do I know if a food is high in added sugar?
Take a look at the label. The ingredients list always starts with the biggest ingredient first.

But watch out for other words used to describe added sugar, such as sucrose, glucose, fructose, maltose, hydrolysed starch and invert sugar, corn syrup and honey. If you see one of these near the top of the list, you know the food is likely to be high in added sugars.

Another way to get an idea of how much sugar is in a food is to have a look for the 'Carbohydrates (of which sugars)' figure on the label. But this figure can't tell you how much is from added sugars, which is the type we should try to cut down on.

10g sugars or more per 100g is **a lot** of sugar 2g sugars or less per 100g is **a little** sugar

If the amount of sugars is between 2g and 10g per 100g, this is a moderate amount.

Sometimes you will only see a figure for total 'Carbohydrates', not for 'Carbohydrates (of which sugars)', which means the figure also includes the carbohydrate from starchy foods.

5. Try to eat less salt – no more that 6g a day
A high salt intake increases the risk of high blood pressure. Most of the salt we eat comes from processed foods so check labels and look for lower salt options in the supermarket and avoid adding too much salt during cooking and at the table.

How do I know if a food is high in salt?
Salt is often listed as sodium on food labels.
Salt = sodium x 2.5.

Use the following as a guide to what is a lot and what is a little salt (or sodium) per 100g food.

This is **a lot** of salt
1.25g salt or more per 100g
0.5g sodium or more per 100g

This is **a little** salt
0.25g salt or less per 100g
0.1g sodium or less per 100g

6. Get active and try and be a healthy weight
Try to be active every day and build up the amount you do. For example, you could try to fit in as much walking as you can into your daily routine. Try to walk at a good pace. It's not a good idea to be either underweight or overweight. Being overweight can lead to health conditions such as heart disease, high blood pressure or diabetes. Being underweight could also affect your health.

7. Drink plenty of water
Drinking plenty of water (6–8 glasses) will make sure you are always well hydrated. Being just 2 % dehydrated can affect mental concentration and 5 % dehydration can affect physical performance. When the weather is warm or when we get active, our bodies need more than this.

8. Don't skip breakfast
Breakfast can help give us the energy we need to face the day, as well as some of the vitamins and minerals we need for good health.

Some people skip breakfast because they think it will help them lose weight. But missing meals doesn't help us lose weight and it isn't good for us, because we can miss out on essential nutrients.

Research shows that eating breakfast can actually help people control their weight. This is probably because when we don't have breakfast we're more likely to get hungry before lunch and snack on foods that are high in fat and sugar, such as biscuits, doughnuts or pastries.

Key point
The Government's eight tips for eating well are:

1. Base your meals on starchy foods

2. Eat lots of fruit and veg

3. Eat more fish

4. Cut down on saturated fat and sugar

5. Try to eat less salt – no more that 6g a day

6. Get active and try and be a healthy weight

7. Drink plenty of water

8. Don't skip breakfast

The link between diet and ill health

The scientific evidence for the relationship between diet and disease is regularly reviewed by expert committees. A person's genes, which they inherit from their parents, influence his or her risk of developing various diseases. Other factors, such as diet, physical activity and smoking, also have an effect on a person's health.

Common health problems linked to diet include:

- a diet high in saturates is recognised as a contributor to heart disease

- excessive amounts of calories above that which is required for activity are a major cause of obesity

- Type 2 diabetes is associated with obesity

- strokes are associated with obesity and high levels of sodium (mainly from salt) in the diet

- cancers such as bowel cancer is linked with inadequate fibre in the diet

- constipation can be due to too little fibre and fluid

- tooth decay (dental caries) can be due to excessive and frequent consumption of sugary foods and drinks.

Strokes

Strokes are related to both high blood pressure and an excessive alcohol intake. High blood pressure is particularly common in people who are overweight and obese. There is also evidence to suggest that the chance of having high blood pressure is greater in people with a high salt intake. The Food Standards Agency considers that reducing the average daily salt intake by one third could reduce strokes by about a third, saving thousands of lives a year. To reduce the risk of having a stroke, people are encouraged to achieve a healthy weight for their height, avoid becoming obese, reduce their salt intake and drink alcohol within sensible limits.

Heart disease

Another example is the risk of heart disease, which is increased by a number of factors including high blood pressure and high levels of cholesterol in the blood. A diet high in saturates can lead to increased levels of cholesterol in the blood. To reduce high blood pressure and, therefore, the risk of heart disease, people are encouraged to maintain a healthy body weight, lower salt intake, avoid high alcohol intakes and have a diet low in saturates. Other advice is to stop smoking, to be more active, to eat plenty of fruit and vegetables and to eat oily fish once a week.

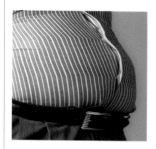

Strokes and heart disease are linked to obesity

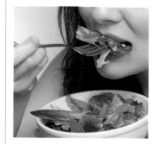

Eating a healthy diet and maintaining a healthy body weight can pay dividends

Obesity

Obesity is a growing problem in the UK, currently 43 % of men and 33 % of women are overweight and 22 % of men and 23 % of women are obese. Obese people also have an increased risk of heart disease, stroke and Type 2 diabetes.

Obesity can be defined using the Body Mass Index (BMI) calculation. The BMI can be calculated as follows:

$$\frac{\text{Weight in kilograms}}{(\text{Height in metres})^2}$$

Example: a woman of height 1.65 metres and weight of 63.6 kilograms.

$$\frac{63.6}{(1.65 \times 1.65)}$$
$$= 23.4$$

Definition for adults:	
below 18.5	underweight
18.5 – 24.9	healthy weight range
25 – 29.9	overweight
above 30	obese

Often charts are used to help assess a person's BMI.

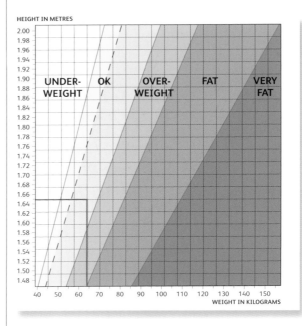

Where a person lays down extra stores of body fat can be important to their health – fat deposited around the waist is the unhealthiest. People who are 'apple shaped', therefore, are at greater risk of health problems associated with obesity than those who are 'pear shaped' (fat deposited around the hips and thighs).

Waist measurements give an indication of obesity – women are encouraged to keep a waist measurement below 31 inches (88cm) and men below 37 inches (94cm) to avoid health problems.

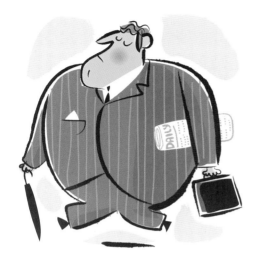

Diabetes

More than one million people are currently diagnosed with diabetes in England and the number continues to grow. Diabetes occurs when the body cannot properly manage the amount of sugar (glucose) that circulates in the blood.

There are two types of diabetes:

Type 1 diabetes – affects younger people and occurs when the pancreas (the gland in the body that produces insulin) ceases to produce insulin. People with Type 1 diabetes need to have injections of insulin plus a diet to control the condition.

Type 2 diabetes – affects older people when the insulin is not as effective in managing blood sugar levels as the fat tissue are resistant to its effect. Therefore people with Type 2 diabetes are usually overweight or obese. People with Type 2 diabetes often only need a diet to control the condition.

Obesity and Type 2 diabetes can be reduced by:

- maintaining a healthy weight
- eating a balanced diet
- increasing physical activity levels.

Key points

- Common health problems, including coronary heart disease, obesity, Type 2 diabetes, strokes, some cancers, constipation and tooth decay can be diet-related.

- The Food Standards Agency considers that reducing the average daily salt intake by one third could reduce strokes by about a third.

- Obesity is a growing problem in the UK and obese people have an increased risk of heart disease, stroke and Type 2 diabetes.

- People who are 'apple shaped' are at greater risk of health problems than those who are 'pear shaped'.

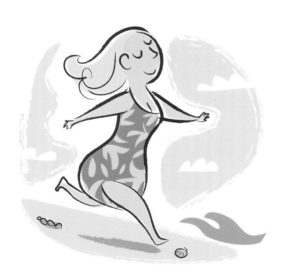

Dietary recommendations

Because of the established links between diet and ill health, the Government makes recommendations about how much fat and saturates, carbohydrate and non-milk extrinsic sugars (NMES), salt and fibre there should be in the average diet. A diet low in saturates, NMES and salt and high in carbohydrates and fibre is regarded as healthy because it is associated with a lower risk of ill health and disease.

Five portions of fruit and vegetables should be eaten each day.

Finally, it is recommended that at least two portions of fish are eaten per week – one of which should be an oily fish such as salmon, pilchards, trout, fresh tuna, herrings and mackerel.

Other dietary recommendations exist for children, pregnant women and other groups of the population (*see* Chapter 4).

Key point

- A diet low in saturates, NMES and salt and high in carbohydrates and fibre is regarded as healthy because it is associated with a lower risk of ill health and disease.

Government dietary recommendations

Percentage daily energy from fat	No more than 35%
Of which, percentage daily energy from saturates	No more than 11%
Percentage daily energy from carbohydrates	At least 50%
Of which, percentage daily energy from NMES	No more than 11%
Grams of salt per day	No more than 6g
Grams of fibre per day	18g

Guideline daily amounts (GDAs)

	Women	Men
Energy (kcal)	2,000	2,500
Fat (g)	70	95
Saturates (g)	20	30
Salt (g)	5	7

Government recommendations for safe alcohol consumption

Men	No more than four units per day
Women	No more than three units per day

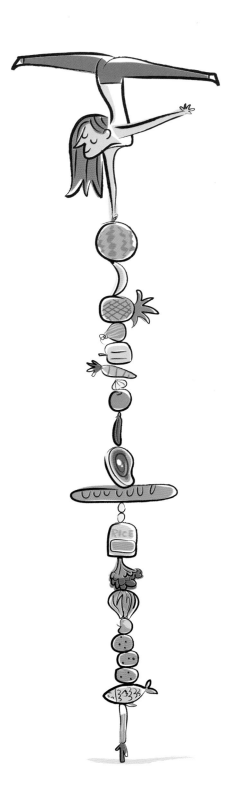

The positive effects of a balanced diet

People who eat a balanced diet not only feel better, but also usually have better health.

Good nutrition can help in preventing disease and obesity by developing eating habits, which are associated with maintaining good health throughout life. For example, for someone obese, only a steady reduction in energy intake – of about 500 kcal (2,100 kJ) per day – and/or increase in physical activity to increase energy expenditure (not sporadic bouts of starvation or exercise) will lead to a weight loss that can be maintained.

A vitamin deficiency will not result from a diet that is lacking in that vitamin for a few days. Nevertheless, the diet is much more likely to contain enough vitamins especially the important antioxidants, if fruit and vegetables are eaten every day than if they are eaten only at infrequent intervals.

Although heart disease will not result from eating the occasional fat-rich meal, it is wise not to include large amounts of fat because it has a high energy value, which will contribute to obesity. Also saturated fat should not be eaten in large amounts every day because of its effect on harmful blood cholesterol levels.

The maintenance of a sensible and regular eating pattern is important for everyone. It is particularly important for those whose needs are high – for example, a pregnant woman, young child or an elderly person. A diet made up of a wide range of different foods so that it is varied and interesting is more likely to be enjoyed.

Key points

- People who eat a balanced diet not only feel better, but also usually have better health.

- Sensible and regular eating patterns are important for everyone.

Tackling diet-related disease in the UK

At present, coronary heart disease and stroke are major causes of early death, accounting for approximately 41,000 deaths each year in people aged below 75 years. In fact the UK has one of the highest rates of heart disease in Western Europe.

In addition, cancer still affects almost every family in the UK at some time. Around two in five people develop cancer during their lifetime and one in four people die from it. Not all cancers are preventable or related to diet but, in many cases, the risks of cancer can be reduced by tackling factors such as diet, smoking and lifestyle. It is estimated that poor diet contributes to around a quarter of all cancers. In particular, low consumption of fruit and vegetables is linked with an increased risk of bowel and stomach cancer.

Successive governments, concerned about the number of people affected by diet-related diseases, have sought to improve the health of the population through various campaigns and initiatives to improve diets and lifestyles.

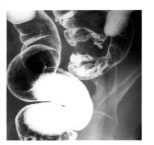

Low consumption of fruit and vegetables is linked to bowel cancer

Key points

- Coronary heart disease and stroke and cancer are major causes of early death.

- Low consumption of fruit and vegetables is linked with an increased risk of bowel and stomach cancer.

- Successive governments have is committed to reducing the number of people affected by diet-related diseases.

Summary

1. No single food contains all the essential nutrients the body needs to be healthy and function efficiently.

2. The eatwell plate is an illustrated guide showing the proportion and types of foods needed to make up a healthy diet.

3. The guide is presented as a dinner plate so it is easy to understand.

4. The plate is divided into five segments representing the proportions of five food groups:

- fruit and vegetables
- bread, rice, potatoes, pasta and other starchy foods
- meat, fish, eggs, beans and other non-dairy sources of protein
- milk and dairy foods
- foods and drinks high in fat and/or sugar.

5. It is not necessary to achieve this balance at each meal, the balance may be achieved over a day or even a week.

6. The Government's eight tips for eating well are:

- Base your meals on starchy foods
- Eat lots of fruit and veg
- Eat more fish
- Cut down on saturated fat and sugar
- Try to eat less salt – no more that 6g a day
- Get active and try and be a healthy weight
- Drink plenty of water
- Don't skip breakfast.

7. Adults are recommended to take no more than 6g of salt per day. Children, much less.

8. Everyone should drink plenty of fluids – being dehydrated can affect mental concentration and physical performance.

9. Common health problems, including coronary heart disease, obesity, Type 2 diabetes, strokes, some cancers, constipation and tooth decay can be diet-related.

10. The Food Standards Agency considers that reducing the average daily salt intake by one third could reduce strokes by about a third.

11. Obesity is a growing problem in the UK and obese people have an increased risk of heart disease, stroke and Type 2 diabetes.

12. People who are 'apple shaped' are at greater risk of health problems than those who are 'pear shaped'.

13. A diet low in saturates, NMESs and salt and high in carbohydrates and fibre is regarded as healthy because it is associated with a lower risk of ill health and disease.

14. People who eat a balanced diet not only feel better, but also usually have better health.

15. Sensible and regular eating patterns are important for everyone.

16. Coronary heart disease and stroke and cancer are major causes of early death.

17. Low consumption of fruit and vegetables is linked with an increased risk of bowel and stomach cancer.

18. Successive governments have committed to reducing the number of people affected by diet-related diseases.

Chapter 4
Nutritional needs and dietary preferences

As you have already seen, people differ in their nutritional needs depending on a number of factors – for example, age, sex, body size and activity level. In addition to nutritional needs, diet is influenced by economic and social factors – for example, cost, access and availability of food, cooking skills and facilities, knowledge, culture and religion. This chapter summarises the different nutritional needs and dietary preferences of certain groups of the population.

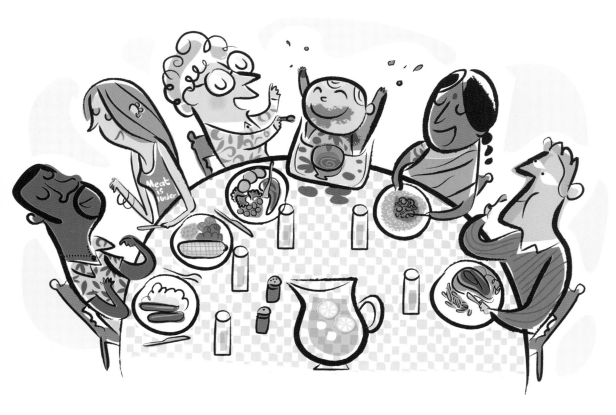

Babies

The first food that babies require is milk. The best source of milk for the baby is the mother's breast milk. This contains all of the nutrients a baby needs in the right amounts. It also provides antibodies from the mother and, therefore, gives the baby extra resistance to diseases. Breastfeeding can help mothers to lose weight gained during pregnancy. So breastfeeding provides benefits to both mother and the child.

For those babies who cannot be breastfed specially made baby milk should be given. These are specially manufactured to contain similar nutrients to breast milk.

Exclusive breastfeeding is recommended for the first six months of a baby's life. Babies should not be weaned (given solid food in addition to milk) until they are around six months old. Breastfeeding (and/or breast milk substitutes, if used) should continue beyond the first six months along with appropriate types and amounts of solid foods.

Waiting until six months to wean helps to minimise the risk of infections and developing allergies. At six months, babies' digestive systems are more developed and their immune systems are stronger. By six months, most babies can learn to chew soft lumpy food, even if they have no teeth, and can quickly progress to finger foods. At six months, babies can eat most types of food, but there are a few that should be avoided until they are one year old – these include, salt, sugar, honey, whole nuts, raw eggs and some types of fish.

If weaning starts before six months, then babies should not be given wheat, gluten or milk. Weaning should not start before four months.

As the baby develops teeth more lumpy foods can be given until, by the age of a year, a child should be eating a wide variety of foods. At the age of a one a child can drink whole milk (during weaning babies should only have whole milk as an ingredient in other foods such as custards). Children need the extra calories from the fat and vitamins A and D that whole milk contains. Semi-skimmed milk can be introduced from the age of two and skimmed milk from five years of age, if preferred.

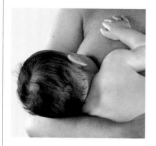

The first food that babies require is milk

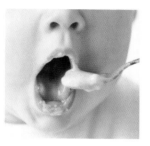

Babies should not be weaned until six months

Key points

- Breast milk contains all of the nutrients a baby needs in the right amounts.

- Exclusive breastfeeding is recommended for the first six months of a baby's life.

- Babies should not be weaned until they are around six months old.

Children

School-aged children grow fast and are very active so energy requirements are high in relation to their body size compared with those of adults. The big appetites of some older children usually reflect a real nutritional need rather than greed. Because of their smaller size compared with adults, and correspondingly smaller stomachs, it is important that young children eat meals that are not too bulky but are packed with nutrients.

Milk, whether whole, semi-skimmed or skimmed, is one of the best sources of calcium, riboflavin and protein. This calcium is particularly important for the development of the skeleton.

Fruit and vegetables should be encouraged for children. Bread, pasta, rice, potatoes and breakfast cereals should be all given as part of a child's diet. Meat, fish, eggs and pulses should also be provided. Whole nuts should not be given to children under five years because of the danger of them choking.

Children should be taught sensible eating habits from an early age – biscuits, sweets, soft drinks, chips and crisps should not displace other foods too often. While children often require snacks between meals, it is better to base these on fruit, bread and plain biscuits rather than foods containing high levels of fat, sugar and/or salt.

Children should be encouraged to clean their teeth twice every day with a fluoride toothpaste.

Foods that may contain a lot of salt – including ready meals, instant noodles, canned beans, ketchups and sauces, sausages, burgers, bacon and salty snacks like potato crisps should be eaten only in moderation. Most foods have labels stating sodium or salt content. As a guide, school-aged children should not consume more than 4g of salt per day (1g of sodium = 2.5g salt). This is only about a small level teaspoonful of salt. The salt intake of younger children should be kept to a minimum so they should not be given salty snacks and foods containing large amounts of salt.

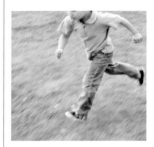

Children grow fast and are very active

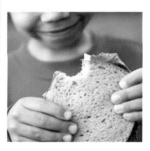

Big appetites usually reflect real nutritional need, not greed

Key points

- Because children grow fast and are very active they have high energy requirements in relation to their body size.

- Children, however, have small stomachs and, so, need to eat meals that are not too bulky and are packed with nutrients.

- Children should be taught sensible eating habits from an early age.

- Eating too many foods containing high levels of fat, sugar and/or salt and fizzy drinks should be avoided.

Adolescents

The nutrient needs of adolescents (teenagers) are higher in many respects than those of any other group. This is because they are still growing and are also at their most active. Healthy adolescents have large appetites and it is important that they should satisfy them with food of a high nutritional value in the form of well-balanced meals rather than by too many snacks containing high levels of fat, sugar or salt.

Obesity among children and young people is increasing and there are concerns that this can lead to the development of health problems in adulthood. It is vital that children are encouraged to eat a wide variety of foods, including fruit and vegetables, and to maintain and develop levels of physical activity to prevent disease in later life.

Key points

- The nutrient needs of adolescents are higher, in many respects, than those of any other group.

- It is important to satisfy large appetites with food of a high nutritional value in the form of well-balanced meals rather than by too many snacks containing high levels of fat, sugar or salt.

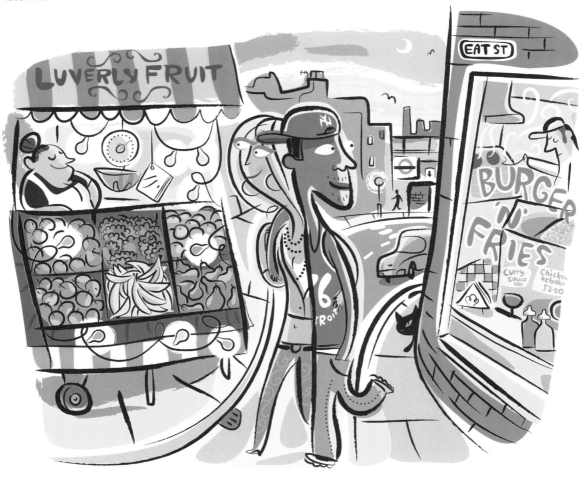

Adults

Many adults in Britain are more likely to be at risk of being over-nourished (consuming too many calories and fat) rather than being under-nourished. In general, healthy, well-balanced diets are high in starchy foods and fruit and vegetables, contain moderate amounts of meat, fish or alternatives and milk and dairy foods, and only small quantities of foods containing fat and sugar.

The starchy carbohydrate from cereal products (including bread, rice and pasta), and from potatoes or other tubers (such as yams), is needed to make sure the diet contains enough energy. These foods will also contribute fibre for bowel health. Sodium intake can be reduced by adding little or no salt at the table and in meal preparation and by choosing reduced-salt ingredients and products.

It is also important to keep alcohol intake within sensible limits:

- 3–4 units/day (men)
- 2–3 units/day (women)

Avoid binge drinking. If you drink too much, try to avoid alcohol for 48 hours.

A unit of alcohol is:

- half a pint of ordinary beer or larger
- a small glass of wine
- a small schooner glass of sherry
- a single 'pub' measure of spirits, such as vodka, gin, whisky, brandy
- half a bottle of most 'alcopop' drinks.

Key points

- A healthy, well-balanced diet for an adult is high in starchy foods and fruit and vegetables, contains moderate amounts of meat, fish or alternatives and milk and dairy foods, and only small quantities of foods containing fat and sugar.
- Avoid binge drinking – if you drink too much, avoid alcohol for 48 hours.

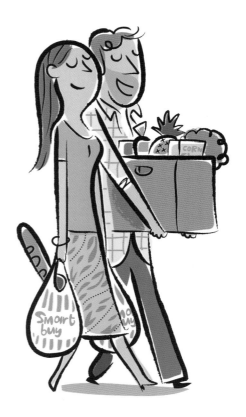

Pregnant and breastfeeding women

A woman's nutritional needs increase during pregnancy and while breastfeeding. This is not only because her diet must provide for the growth and development of her child, but also because other changes occur in the woman's body. These include the laying down of new tissues – such as an increased development of the breasts and womb tissues – as well as an increased blood volume. Extra fat is deposited during pregnancy to provide an energy store to meet the additional demands of the growing foetus and the breastfed infant.

It is most important that the pregnant woman's diet contains sufficient energy, protein, iron, calcium, folate (folic acid) and vitamins C and D for building the baby's muscular tissues, bones and teeth, and for the formation of haemoglobin. This is the red-coloured substance in red blood cells, which carries oxygen around the body to all cells. If not, the woman's own stores of nutrients may be reduced. In practice, most of the extra nutrients needed by a woman during pregnancy will be obtained simply by satisfying the appetite with a good mixed diet – including plenty of starchy carbohydrate foods, fruit and vegetables, dairy products, and meat, fish or its alternatives.

Pregnant women should avoid eating shark, swordfish and marlin and limit the amount of tuna they eat to no more than two tuna steaks a week (weighing about 140g cooked or 170g raw) or four medium-size cans of tuna a week (with a drained weight of about 140g per can). This is because of the levels of mercury in these fish. At high levels, mercury can harm a baby's developing nervous system.

Pregnant women should have no more than two portions of oily fish a week. Oily fish includes fresh tuna (not canned tuna, which does not count as oily fish), mackerel, sardines and trout.

Eating fish is good for a pregnant woman's health and the development of her baby, so she should still aim to eat at least two portions of fish a week, including one portion of oily fish.

Extra folate, before and during early pregnancy, is recommended for all women to decrease the risk of occurrence of neural tube defects in babies. All women of childbearing age are advised to take a daily supplement of 0.4mg of folic acid as well as eating folate-rich foods (see the table of vitamins in Chapter 1). These supplements should be continued for the first 12 weeks of pregnancy. Those who have already given birth to a child with neural tube defects should take and increased amount (4mg) of folic acid each day. Pregnant women also need to take supplements containing 10 mcg of vitamin D each day.

Pregnant women are, however, advised *not* to take supplements containing vitamin A or eat foods (particularly liver and foods containing liver like pates and faggots) that may be rich in vitamin A, except on the advice of their doctor, due to the possible risk of birth defects. Some women may be advised to take iron supplements by their doctor to prevent anemia.

A number of foods should be avoided during pregnancy to reduce the risk of food poisoning – for example, unpasteurised soft cheeses and mould ripened cheeses, which can contain Listeria.

Excessive alcohol intake should also be avoided during pregnancy. Some pregnant women may choose to avoid alcohol altogether.

During breastfeeding extra energy, protein, iron, calcium, phosphorus and vitamins are needed as well as extra fluid to enable the mother to produce breast milk.

Key points

- A woman's nutritional needs increase during pregnancy and while breastfeeding.

- Most of the extra nutrients needed by a woman during pregnancy will be supplied by a good mixed diet.

- Eating fish is good for a pregnant woman's health and the development of her baby, so she should aim to eat at least two portions of fish a week, including one portion of oily fish.

- Folic acid supplements before and during early pregnancy are recommended for all women to decrease the risk of occurrence of neural tube defects in babies.

- A number of foods should be avoided during pregnancy to reduce the risk of food poisoning.

- Extra energy, protein, iron, calcium, phosphorus and vitamins are needed as well as extra fluid to enable women to produce breast milk.

Older people

As age progresses and body weight and energy expenditure decreases, people tend to eat less and hence may find it difficult to satisfy all the nutrient requirements. It is important, therefore, that older people are encouraged to remain active and to maintain a good energy intake unless they are obese. They should also have foods that are concentrated sources of protein, vitamins and minerals. A healthy weight can be more readily maintained and recovery from illness or injury will be more rapid if older people are also encouraged to eat a healthy well-balanced diet and take plenty of gentle exercise.

Older people also benefit from eating plenty of fruit and vegetables (these may be better stewed, juiced or pureed if the person experiences problems with eating due to a lack of teeth). Fruit and vegetables are sometimes lacking in the diets of older people, but they are important in order to prevent vitamin C deficiency. Foods rich in fibre can also help to prevent constipation, which is common in elderly people.

Good dietary sources of vitamin D such as margarine, eggs or oily fish (such as sardines, mackerel) are important in the diet (*see* table of vitamins in Chapter 1). Everyone over the age of 65, but especially those who do not go outside in the sunlight because they are completely housebound, should consider taking a daily vitamin D supplement.

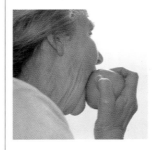

A healthy diet can help to promote health and recovery

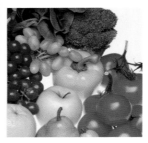

Older people need to ensure their diets provide plenty of vitamins C and D and fibre

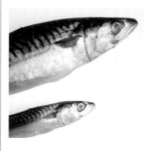

Key point

- A well-balanced diet and plenty of gentle exercise can help the older person to maintain a healthy weight and promote recovery following an illness or injury.

Slimmers

As already stated, being overweight or obese is a significant problem for a large number of people. Planning a slimming diet is a matter of individual preference. Essentially, energy intake needs to be cut down by 500–1000 kcal (2,092–4,182 kJ) per day to achieve a weekly weight loss of 0.5–1.0kg (1–2lb). Other nutrients should still reach recommended levels.

It is best cut out high-fat and high-sugar foods – such as, cakes, sweets, preserves, biscuits and some puddings – as well as alcohol, as these tend to be sources of energy rather than nutrients. Low- or reduced-fat and reduced sugar products sometimes called 'light', which are now readily available, can be substituted for high-fat and high-sugar foods. Slimmers should be aware, however, that some low-fat products may contain high levels of sugar.

Fat can be trimmed from meat, and foods can be boiled or grilled rather than fried or served with creamy sauces and pastry. Foods high in water (such as fruit and vegetables) or fibre (such as bread, cereals, pasta, rice, and oats) can give feelings of fullness and so reduce the desire for more food.

The key to successful weight loss is to cut down on food intake and increase activity levels.

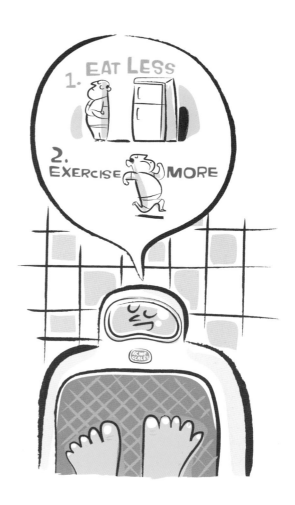

Key points

- Being overweight or obese is a significant problem for a large number of people.

- The key to successful weight loss is to cut down on food intake and increase activity levels.

Vegetarians and vegans

Vegetarians do not eat meat or fish, but do eat some animal products – such as milk, cheese and eggs. In general, the nutritional value of vegetarian diets is very similar to that of mixed (omnivorous) diets, but those based largely on vegetables, having a high water and fibre content, may be rather bulky and lower in energy.

Vegans eat no foods of animal origin at all. Human nutrient requirements, with the exception of vitamin B_{12}, can be met by a diet composed entirely of plant foods. However vegan diets must be carefully planned using a wide selection of foods. A mixture of plant proteins derived from cereals, peas, beans and nuts will provide enough protein of good quality, but special care is needed to ensure that sufficient energy, calcium, iron, zinc, riboflavin, vitamin B_{12} and vitamin D are also available. Yeast extract is a good source of some of the B vitamins, including vitamin B_{12}, that are otherwise found mainly in foods of animal origin.

In extreme vegan diets, such as Zen macrobiotic diets where little but wholegrain cereals are eaten, intakes of calcium, iron, vitamin B_{12} and vitamin C are likely to be too low for health.

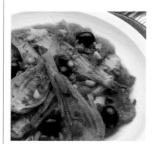

The nutritional value of a vegetarian diet is similar to a mixed diet

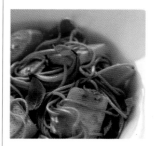

Vegan diets must be carefully planned using a wide selection of foods

Key points

- In general, the nutritional value of vegetarian diets is very similar to that of mixed (omnivorous) diets.

- Vegan diets must be carefully planned using a wide selection of foods to ensure that sufficient energy, calcium, iron, zinc, riboflavin, vitamin B_{12} and vitamin D are provided.

Ethnic minority groups

In general, the traditional diets of ethnic minority groups provide adequate nourishment. The table below shows some of the dietary restrictions and practices of some religious and ethnic minority groups.

Dietary restrictions

Group	Dietary restriction	Other dietary practices
Hindus	No beef Fish rarely eaten No alcohol Period of fasting common	Mostly vegetarian
Muslims	No pork Halal meat* No shellfish No alcohol	Regular fasting, including Ramadan for one month
Sikhs	No beef Animal for meat must be killed by 'one blow to the head' No alcohol	Generally less rigid eating restrictions than Hindus or Muslims
Jews	No pork Kosher meat** Separation of meat and dairy Only fish with scales and fins may be eaten	
Rastafarians	No animal products except milk may be consumed Foods must be I-tal or be alive Foods must be organic No processed or canned food No salt to be added No coffee or alcohol	

*Animals slaughtered and prepared in accordance with Shari'ah law
**Animals slaughtered and prepared in accordance with Jewish law

Recent immigrants to the UK, who have may difficulty adapting their traditional diets and customs to local circumstances, may have special dietary problems. In particular, Asian vegetarian groups may have very low intakes of vitamin D – a problem sometimes compounded by lack of exposure to sunlight (especially by women and children) because of customs of dress and a tendency to remain indoors. Without vitamin D to aid calcium absorption, bone disorders can develop. Good sources of vitamin D should, therefore, be included in the diet and vitamin supplements may be necessary. Iron deficiency (anemia) – characterised by tiredness, paleness and poor wound healing – may occur among women and children, particularly in the Asian community, whose diets consist mainly of vegetables and cereals.

A genetic predisposition to diabetes is linked to ethnic background. People from African-Caribbean or Asian backgrounds living in the UK are four to five times more likely to have Type 2 diabetes than white members of the population.

People with diabetes

Diabetes is a metabolic disorder that reduces the ability of the body to control the amount of glucose in the blood. Glucose in the blood provides cells in the body with energy.

It is important for people with diabetes to avoid large fluctuations in blood glucose by controlling blood glucose levels through the use of medication (injections of insulin) and/or diet. Obesity reduces the body's ability to metabolise glucose and can, therefore, worsen diabetic control. Generally, people with diabetes should eat diets similar to those recommended for other adults.

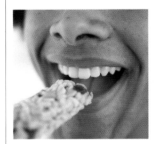

Type 2 diabetes is linked to ethnic background

Key points

- In general, the traditional diets of ethnic minority groups provide adequate nourishment.

- Some dietary and cultural restrictions and practices of religious and ethnic minority groups may result in specific nutritional problems.

Food intolerance and allergy

There are people who have to follow special diets for various medical reasons – this includes people with gluten intolerance (coeliac disease) or lactose intolerance. Such intolerances are considered to be medical problems rather than nutritional ones.

Food allergy is a specific form of food intolerance that involves the body's immune system. A small proportion of the population is affected by food allergies that cause individuals to experience an allergic reaction to foods that are harmless for most other people. Food allergy symptoms are varied and range from being mild to potentially fatal. Because food allergies can be life threatening it is very important that anybody working with food intended for consumption by others is allergy aware.

Foods that can trigger an allergic reaction

There are many foods that can cause an allergic reaction – those listed below, however, are responsible for 90 % of allergic reactions within the UK:

- celery
- cereals containing gluten (including wheat, rye, barley and oats)
- crustaceans (including prawns, crabs and lobsters)
- eggs
- fish
- lupin
- milk
- molluscs (including mussels and oysters)
- mustard
- nuts (including Brazil nuts, hazelnuts, almonds and walnuts)
- peanuts (groundnuts or monkey nuts)
- sesame seeds
- soya
- sulphur dioxide or sulphites.

Many allergies start in childhood, but whereas some can be lifelong – such as, allergy to peanuts and nuts – some can be outgrown before school age, this is typical for reactions to milk and eggs. Allergy to a food can, however, start at any age – for example, reaction to shellfish more often develops in adults. Food allergies affect about 1–2 % of children and less than 1 % of adults, nevertheless, reactions can be extremely serious.

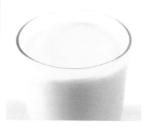

Foods that can trigger an allergic reaction include milk, eggs and peanuts

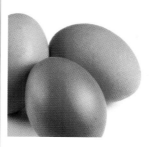

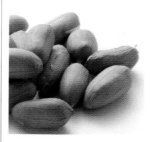

Anaphylaxis

Anaphylaxis is a reaction that can be life threatening, it can occur as an allergic response to a food. Anaphylaxis can cause some or all of the following symptoms:

- swelling of the throat or mouth
- difficulty swallowing or speaking
- difficulty breathing
- skin rash or flushing
- abdominal cramps, nausea, vomiting
- sudden weakness
- collapse and unconsciousness.

If these symptoms occur:

- call 999 and ask for an ambulance
- say that you think the person has anaphylaxis (anna-fill-axis)
- stay with the person until help arrives.

It is very important that people who handle, prepare and/or serve food understand how to control the risks posed by food allergies. If you do not know what ingredients are in a food or product, always seek advice, *NEVER* guess. Be aware that although a food may not contain a certain ingredient it may still cause a reaction if it has been contaminated by the ingredient at some point in the process of preparation or production.

Legislation in the UK requires that consumers are given comprehensive ingredient listing information on pre-packaged food to make it easier for people with food allergies to identify ingredients they need to avoid.

The 14 most common food allergens (listed on p. 49) must be indicated by reference to the source allergen whenever they, or ingredients made from them, are used at any level in pre-packed foods, including alcoholic drinks.

The presence of the allergen must be clear to the consumer. For example the label must make it clear that caseins/caseinates and whey products are derived from milk, lecithin from soya and flavourings must include source ingredients – that is, flavouring (contains almond).

Legislation covers only ingredients added intentionally and not traces that may be present due to cross-contamination.

Some products might be labelled e.g. 'free from' or 'may contain' in relation to certain ingredients like nuts, wheat and milk.

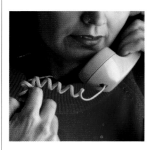

If you think someone has anaphylaxis, call for an ambulance

Key points

- A small proportion of the population is affected by food allergies that cause individuals to experience an allergic reaction to foods that are harmless for most other people.

- Food allergy symptoms are varied and range from being mild to potentially fatal.

- Foods known to cause and allergic reaction include cereals containing gluten, shellfish, eggs, fish, peanuts, etc.

- It is very important that people who handle, prepare and/or serve food understand how to control the risks posed by food allergies.

Summary

1. Breast milk contains all of the nutrients a baby needs in the right amounts.

2. Exclusive breastfeeding is recommended for the first six months of a baby's life.

3. Babies should not be weaned until they are around six months old.

4. Because children grow fast and are very active they have high energy requirements in relation to their body size.

5. Children, however, have small stomachs and, so, need to eat meals that are not too bulky and are packed with nutrients.

6. Children should be taught sensible eating habits from an early age.

7. Consuming large quantities of foods and drinks containing high levels of fat, sugar and/or salt and fizzy drinks should be avoided.

8. The nutrient needs of adolescents are higher, in many respects, than those of any other group.

9. It is important to satisfy large appetites satisfy them with food of a high nutritional value in the form of well-balanced meals rather than by too many snacks containing high levels of fat, sugar or salt.

10. A healthy, well-balanced diet for an adult is high in starchy foods and fruit and vegetables, contains moderate amounts of meat, fish or alternatives and milk and dairy foods, and only small quantities of foods and drinks containing fat and/or sugar.

11. Avoid binge drinking – if you drink too much, avoid alcohol for 48 hours.

12. A woman's nutritional needs increase during pregnancy and while breastfeeding.

13. Most of the extra nutrients needed by a woman during pregnancy will be supplied by a good mixed diet.

14. Eating fish is good for a pregnant woman's health and the development of her baby, so she should aim to eat at least two portions of fish a week, including one portion of oily fish.

15. Folic acid supplements before and during early pregnancy are recommended for all women to decrease the risk of occurrence of neural tube defects in babies.

16. A number of foods should be avoided during pregnancy to reduce the risk of food poisoning.

17. Extra energy, protein, iron, calcium, phosphorus and vitamins are needed as well as extra fluid to enable women to produce breast milk.

18. A well-balanced diet and plenty of gentle exercise can help the older person to maintain a healthy weight and promote recovery following an illness or injury.

19. Being overweight or obese is a significant problem for a large number of people.

20. The key to successful weight loss is to cut down on food intake and increase activity levels.

21. In general, the nutritional value of vegetarian diets is very similar to that of mixed (omnivorous) diets.

22. Vegan diets must be carefully planned using a wide selection of foods to ensure that sufficient energy, calcium, iron, zinc, riboflavin, vitamin B_{12} and vitamin D are provided.

23. In general, the traditional diets of ethnic minority groups provide adequate nourishment.

24. Some dietary and cultural restrictions and practices of religious and ethnic minority groups may result in specific nutritional problems.

25. A small proportion of the population is affected by food allergies that cause individuals to experience an allergic reaction to foods that are harmless for most other people.

26. Food allergy symptoms are varied and range from being mild to potentially fatal.

27. Foods known to cause and allergic reaction include celery, cereals containing gluten (including wheat, rye, barley and oats), crustaceans (including prawns, crabs and lobsters), eggs, fish, lupin, milk, molluscs (including mussels and oysters), mustard, nuts (including Brazil nuts, hazelnuts, almonds and walnuts), peanuts (groundnuts or monkey nuts), sesame seeds, soya and sulphur dioxide or sulphites.

28. It is very important that people who handle, prepare and/or serve food understand how to control the risks posed by food allergies.

Chapter 5
Catering in institutions and other settings

At various times of life the food received in institutions plays an important role in the diet of individuals. Often caterers may be faced with a challenge to provide a balanced diet within a strict budget – this type of catering is often referred to as 'cost sector catering'. As more and more people, in general, are eating food prepared outside of the home, people working in the food industry can have a major influence on the nation's diet and have a key role in helping achieve these government targets to improve the nation's health, by offering customers the choice of healthier food options.

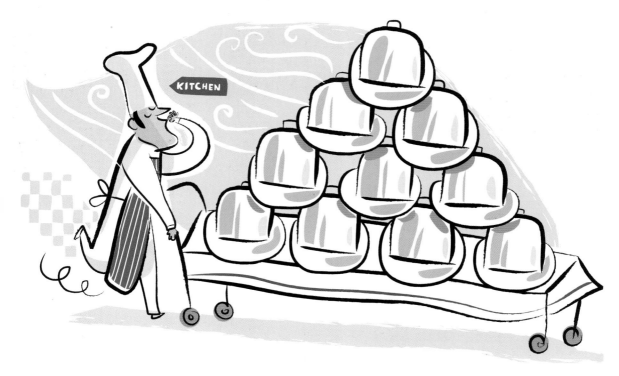

Hospitals

Hospital caterers have an opportunity to promote healthy eating habits amongst patients and staff. However, healthy eating principles are not applicable to all patients. For some patients, the primary aim should be to ensure that they are adequately nourished to allow them to get well and this may mean sometimes providing high-fat and high-sugar foods just to tempt them to eat.

Food in hospitals should be considered as part of the treatment and care of a patient. Hospital caterers can play a part in improving the nutritional status of patients who come into hospital undernourished. These patients need foods that are high in energy and nutrients to aid recovery. Social, cultural and religious requirements must also be considered as familiar food is more likely to be acceptable to someone who is ill. This presents a real challenge for caterers.

Guidelines for hospital food provide standards appropriate for the general hospital population and standards for specific patient groups. There are menus suitable for patients who:

- are children
- require food of a modified consistency such as soft or puree food
- require high energy food
- require cultural and religious dishes.

There are guidelines on a range of catering issues, including menu planning, food distribution, snacks and service on wards as well as a database of seasonal recipes.

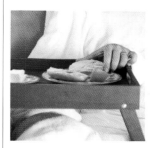

Patients may need to be tempted to eat

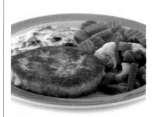

Foods that are high in energy and nutrients may aid recovery

Key points

- Hospital caterers have an opportunity to promote healthy eating habits amongst patients and staff.

- Food in hospitals should be considered as part of the treatment and care of a patient.

- Hospital caterers can play a part in improving the nutritional status of patients who come into hospital undernourished.

- Guidelines for hospital food provide standards appropriate for the general hospital population and standards for specific patient groups.

Schools

The school years are a good time to promote healthy eating and, thereby, contribute to children's health, ability to learn and future well being. For many pupils the meal they eat at school is the main meal of the day. Providing food that pupils will enjoy and that is healthy can be a challenge for school caterers. School meals also need to allow for the different cultural and religious requirements.

Since the removal of the obligation, through the 1980 Education Act, to provide meals to school-children except to those who were entitled to a free school meal, much concern has been expressed about the nutritional content of school meals and about the diets of schoolchildren in general.

There are two sets of standards for school lunches: food-based standards and nutrient-based standards.

Food-based standards for lunches

The food-based standards for school lunches define the types of food that should be offered in a school lunch and their frequency and are summarised as follows:

1. At least two portions of fruit and vegetables must be provided per day per pupil – at least one should be salad or vegetables and at least one should be fruit.

2. Oily fish must be provided at least once every three weeks.

3. Manufactured meat products may be served occasionally as part of school lunches provided that they meet specific standards for minimum meat content and do not contain any prohibited offal.

4. Bread should be available on a daily basis.

5. Meals should not contain more than two deep-fried items per week.

6. The only drinks available should be: plain water (still or fizzy), skimmed or semi-skimmed milk, pure fruit juices, yogurt or milk drinks (with less than 5 % added sugar), drinks made from combinations of any of the preceding four (e.g. smoothies), low-calorie hot chocolate, tea and coffee – artificial sweeteners may only be used in yogurt or milk drinks, or combinations containing yogurt or milk. The School Food Trust encourages the provision of unsweetened and additive-free drinks wherever possible.

7. Free, fresh drinking water should be provided at all times.

8. Table salt should not be made available and condiments should only be available in sachets.

9. Confectionary and chocolate (excluding cocoa powder used in chocolate cakes, or low calorie hot drinking chocolate) must not be available. The only savoury snacks available should be nuts and seeds with no added salt or sugar. However, food handlers should be aware of nut allergies (see www.allergyinschools.org.uk).

Nutrient-based standards for lunches

The nutrient-based standards set out the proportion of nutrients that children and young people should receive from an average school lunch.

There are 14 nutrient-based standards. The average school lunch should provide 30 % of a pupil's daily energy requirement, which will vary depending on age, body size, metabolism and physical activity, so the standard for energy is based on an average requirement. The remaining 13 nutrients have either maximum standards or minimum standards.

The table below shows the amount of energy the average school lunch should provide. Whilst it shows the maximum amounts of fat, saturated fat, non-milk extrinsic sugars (NMES) and sodium allowed, it shows the minimum amounts of carbohydrate, protein, fibre, vitamin A, vitamin C, folate, calcium, iron and zinc that should be present.

Standards for food other than lunches

The regulations regarding all school food other than lunches state that:

1. No confectionary may be sold in schools.

2. No bagged savoury snacks other than nuts and seeds (without added salt or sugar) may be sold in schools.

3. A variety of fruit and vegetables should be available.

4. Pupils must have easy access to fresh drinking water – preferably this should be chilled and should be located so that pupils do not have to go to the lavatory to access it.

5. The only other drinks available will be plain water (still or fizzy), skimmed or semi-skimmed milk, pure fruit juices, yogurt or milk drinks (with less than 5 % added sugar), drinks made from combinations of any of the preceding four (e.g. smoothies), low-calorie hot chocolate, tea and coffee.

Scotland, Wales and Northern Ireland have their own standards for lunches and food other than lunches.

Nutrient-based standards

Nutrient	Primary	Secondary
Energy (kcal))	530 ± 5 %	646 ± 5 %
Carbohydrate (g)	min 70.6	min 86.1
Non-milk extrinsic sugars (NMES) (g)	max 15.5	max 18.9
Fat (g)	max 20.6	max 25.1
Saturated fat (g)	max 6.5	max 7.9
Protein (g)	min 7.5	min 13.3
Fibre (g)	min 4.2	min 5.2
Sodium (mg)	max 499	max 714
Vitamin A (µg)	min 175	min 245
Vitamin C (mg)	min 10.5	min 14
Folate (µg)	min 53	min 70
Calcium (mg)	min 193	min 350
Iron (mg)	min 3.0	min 5.2
Zinc (mg)	min 2.5	min 3.3

Figures are based on requirements for mixed sex secondary schools.

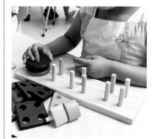

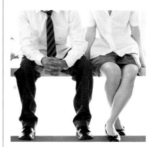

There are compulsory nutritional standards for nursery, primary and secondary school meals

In addition, the Government has introduced a duty to provide paid meals on request for all school pupils over the age of five and for full-time pupils under five. Guidance is given on the nutritional standards, putting together a healthy menu, different cooking methods and how nutritional standards should be monitored, along with case studies and example menus. A whole school approach to nutrition is also encouraged with the involvement of nutrition as part of the curriculum, with vending, breakfast clubs, tuck shops and after-school clubs also being involved.

Separate regulations in Scotland, Wales and Northern Ireland have been produced or are in the process of being developed.

The National School Fruit and Vegetable Scheme provides all 4–6 year olds in infant, primary and special schools in England with a free piece of fruit or vegetable on each school day. Similar initiatives to encourage healthy eating among school children are being developed in other parts of the UK.

The Caroline Walker Trust provides information about health and good nutrition for those catering for children. This includes recipes, help with menu planning and ideas for different ethnic groups.

Key points

- The school years are a good time to promote healthy eating and, thereby, contribute to children's health, ability to learn and future well being.

- Providing food that pupils will enjoy and that is healthy can be a challenge for school caterers.

- There are compulsory nutrient-based and food-based standards for meals in schools and also compulsory standards for all school food other than meals.

Older people in residential care and community meals

A healthy diet is just as important for older people to help maximise good health into old age and to aid recovery from illness.

Many older people in the community rely on the provision of appropriate food for their well-being from services such as Meals on Wheels, luncheon clubs and day centres, as do those in residential care or nursing homes. Some older people suffer from circumstances that can result in a poor food intake. These include poverty and loneliness, poor appetite (due to illness or medication), a declining sense of smell, a lack of interest in food because of depression or bereavement, or difficulties in eating (such as poor teeth) or preparing food (due to arthritis). As a result many elderly people are undernourished or underweight, and in old age this poses a greater risk to health than being overweight.

People become less active as they get older and so their energy needs fall, but requirements for essential nutrients such as vitamins and minerals do not differ greatly from those of younger adults. Older people should, therefore, consume a balanced diet containing nutrient dense foods with adequate vitamins and minerals as well as protein and fibre.

In England and Wales, national minimum standards exist for care homes for older people. Meeting these standards is a core requirement for all care homes providing accommodation, nursing and personal care for older people. Some of the standards relate to food and food provision, which includes specifications about the type of food that is acceptable, when it should be eaten, the appropriate number of meals per day and the timing throughout the day.

Specifically, the standards state that:

- A registered person ensures that service users receive a varied, appealing, wholesome and nutritious diet that is suited to individual assessed and recorded requirements and that meals are taken in congenial settings at flexible times.

- Each service user is offered three full meals each day (at least one of which must be cooked) at intervals of not more than five hours.

- Hot and cold drinks and snacks are available at all times and are offered regularly. A snack meal should be offered in the evening and the interval between this and breakfast the following morning should be no more than 12 hours.

- Food, including liquefied meals, is presented in a manner that is attractive and appealing in terms of texture, flavour and appearance, in order to maintain appetite and nutrition.

- Special therapeutic diets and feeds are provided when advised by health care and dietetic staff, including adequate provision of calcium and vitamin D, the government advises that adults over 65 who do not have adequate exposure to sunlight should take a 10 mcg daily vitamin D supplement..

- Religious and cultural dietary needs are catered for as agreed at admission and recorded in the care plan and food for special occasions is available.

- A registered person ensures that there is a menu (changed regularly) offering choice of meals in written and other formats to suit the capacities of all service users that is given, read or explained to the service users.

- A registered person ensures that mealtimes are unhurried with service users being given sufficient time to eat.

- Staff are ready to offer assistance in eating where necessary, discreetly, sensitively and individually, while independent eating is encouraged as long as possible.

Nutrient- and food-based guidance is given is support of the standards and example menus have been produced.

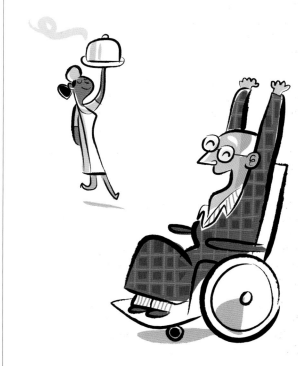

Key points

- Poverty and loneliness, a declining sense of smell, a lack of interest in food because of depression or bereavement, or difficulties in eating or preparing food can affect the appetite of elderly people.

- In old people, being undernourished or underweight poses a greater risk to health than being overweight.

- In England and Wales, national minimum standards exist for care homes for older people. Some of the standards relate to food and food provision, which includes specifications about the type of food that is acceptable, when it should be eaten, the appropriate number of meals per day and the timing throughout the day.

- Nutrient and food-based guidance has been produced in support of the national minimum standards along with example menus.

Prisons and custodial settings

The majority of individuals in prison or custodial settings are young men, but prisoners also include elderly individuals as well as women who may be pregnant or breastfeeding a baby. The prison population is also culturally and religiously diverse.

Periods of custodial care can provide opportunities for promoting a healthy diet and lifestyle, which includes nutrition. The caterers in the HM Prison Service have clearly identified guidelines on all aspects of nutrition and diet in the form of the *Prison Service Catering Manual* (PSO 5000).

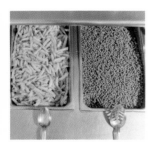

Custodial care can provide an opportunity for promoting a healthy diet

Catering for health

Encouraging people to eat a better diet can help protect against a number of health problems. As more and more people are eating food prepared outside of the home, people working in the food industry can have a major influence on the nation's diet and have a key role in helping the Government achieve these targets, by offering customers the choice of healthier food options. The Food Standards Agency and the Department of Health have produced a guide entitled *Catering for Health* (FSA, 2000) for teaching healthier catering practices.

The key to healthier catering is to:
- make small changes to best-selling items
- increase the amount of starchy foods
- increase the amount of fruit and vegetables
- increase the fibre content of dishes, where practical and acceptable
- reduce fat in traditional recipes
- change the type of fat used
- select healthier ways to prepare dishes
- be moderate in the use of sugar and salt.

Key actions to achieve these goals include:
- make starchy foods (e.g. rice, pasta, bread and potatoes) a main part of most meals
- offer a good selection of fruit and incorporate it into dishes, where practical and acceptable
- offer fibre-rich varieties of breads and cereals
- include plenty of pulses and vegetables in dishes
- use lower fat cooking methods and ingredients
- reduce the amount and alter the types of fat used in food preparation
- use fewer fats that contain a high proportion of saturates by substituting these with fats and oils that have a higher content of unsaturates
- use salt and salty foods in moderation
- add sugar in moderation.

Some practical tips based on the Catering for Health Guide can be found on the information sheets provided with this book.

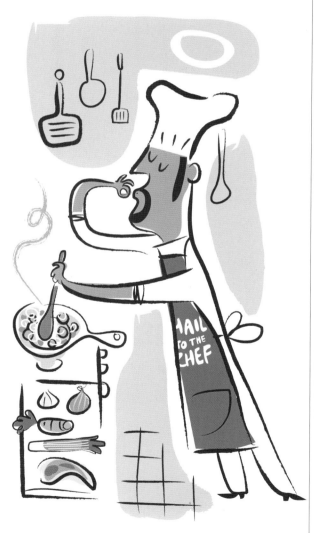

Summary

1. Hospital caterers have an opportunity to promote healthy eating habits amongst patients and staff.

2. Food in hospitals should be considered as part of the treatment and care of a patient.

3. Hospital caterers can play a part in improving the nutritional status of patients who come into hospital undernourished.

4. Guidelines for hospital food provide standards appropriate for the general hospital population and standards for specific patient groups.

5. The school years are a good time to promote healthy eating and, thereby, contribute to children's health, ability to learn and future well being.

6. Providing food that pupils will enjoy and that is healthy can be a challenge for school caterers.

7. There are compulsory nutrient-based and food-based standards for meals in schools and also compulsory standards for all school food other than meals.

8. Poverty and loneliness, a declining sense of smell, a lack of interest in food because of depression or bereavement, or difficulties in eating or preparing food can affect the appetite of elderly people.

9. In old people, being undernourished or underweight poses a greater risk to health than being overweight.

10. In England and Wales, national minimum standards exist for care homes for older people. Some of the standards relate to food and food provision, which includes specifications about the type of food that is acceptable, when it should be eaten, the appropriate number of meals per day and the timing throughout the day.

Index

Editor: Mabel Blades
Design: www.red-stone.com
Illustration: Ned Jolliffe

Photography: 4T (Nancy Rockwell/Digital Vision/Getty Images), 4B (James
Woodson/ Digital Vision/Getty Images), 6T (Digital Vision/ Getty Images),
6M (Maximilian Stock Ltd/Anthony Blake Photo Library), 6B (Andy Crawford/ Getty
Images), 7T (Joerg Lehmann/Getty Images), 7B (davies & starr/Photodisc Red/Getty
Images), 9T (Foodcollection/Getty Images), 9M (Foodcollection/ Getty Images),
9B (Foodcollection/Getty Images), 13T (Tim Hill/Anthony Blake Photo Library),
13M (David Buffington/Photodisc Green/Getty Images), 13B (Graham Kirk/Anthony
Blake Photo Library), 14 (Nino Mascardi/Getty Images), 17 (ATW Photography/Anthony
Blake Photo Library), 19T (Robert Lawson/Anthony Blake Photo Library), 19M (Luzia
Ellert/Getty Images), 19B (Bear Images/ Anthony Blake Photo Library), 29 (David
McGlynn/Getty Images), 31T (GSO Images/Getty Images), 31B (Sarma Ozols/Getty
Images), 36 (Zephyr/ Science Photo Library), 39T (Helen McArdle/ Science Photo
Library), 39B (Jamie Grill/Getty Images), 40T (Andersen Ross/Photodisc Green/Getty
Images), 40B (Richard Schultz/Getty Images), 44T (John Slater/Photodisc Red/ Getty
Images), 44M (davies & starr/Getty Images), 44B (Isabelle Rozenbaum & Frederic
Cirou/PhotoAlto/Getty Images), 46T (Martin Brigdale/Anthony Blake Photo Library),
46B (Joy Skipper/Anthony Blake Photo Library), 48 (Stockdisc/ Stockdisc Premium/Getty
Images), 49T (Graham Day/Anthony Blake Photo Library), 49M (Joff Lee/Anthony Blake
Photo Library), 49B (FoodCollection/ Punchstock), 50 (David Buffington/ Photodisc
Green/Getty Images), 53T (PNC/ Photodisc Red/Getty Images), 53B (Crown copyright
material is reproduced with the permission of the Controller of HMSO and Queen's
Printer for Scotland), 55T (BananaStock/Imagestate), 55B (Tom Merton/Photodisc
Red/Getty Images), 58 (Baerbel Schmidt/Getty Images).

Stock: Cocoon Silk 50, 50 % recycled and 50 % FSC certified ECF pulp

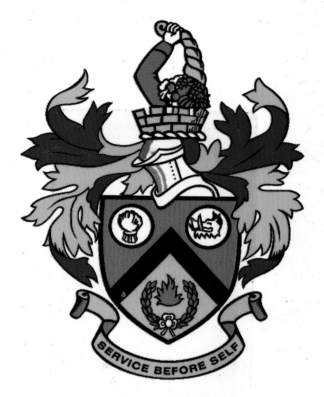

UCB
University College Birmingham

Library
Summer Row
Birmingham
B3 1JB
Tel: 0121 243 0055.
www.ucb.ac.uk